THE MENOPAUSE QUESTION ANSWERED

A NURSE PRACTITIONER'S GUIDE

NAVIGATE HORMONAL CHANGES EASILY, LOSE WEIGHT, SLEEP WELL & NATURALLY CONTROL HOT FLASHES TO IMPROVE OVERALL QUALITY OF LIFE

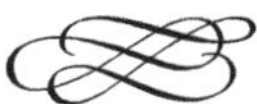

JUDETH BEVERLY, CRNP

TABLE OF CONTENTS

INTRODUCTION

Picture this: Sarah, a vibrant professional in her late 40s, suddenly finds herself struggling with overwhelming fatigue, hot flashes that turn meetings into sweat-soaked challenges, and a memory that seems to have taken an extended vacation. Her once-restful nights now feel like battlegrounds of tossing, turning, and waking up drenched in sweat. It's not just physical; it's impacting her work, her relationships, and her sense of self.

If you're nodding along, feeling Sarah's frustrations, you're not alone. Menopause is a transformative journey that can leave even the most resilient women feeling lost and overwhelmed. The symptoms—ranging from hot flashes, mood swings, and sleep disturbances to weight gain and memory fog—can feel like an unrelenting storm, disrupting the smooth sail of life.

You picked this book not just because of its title but because something resonates deep within you. Maybe it was the night sweats that jolted you awake one too many times or the frustrating memory lapses that made you forget an important meeting. Perhaps it was the sudden weight gain despite your best efforts or the emotional rollercoaster that was leaving you exhausted.

What this book promises is more than just information; it's a roadmap back to yourself. You'll discover shortcuts to reduce your symptoms, regain control of your body and mind, and rediscover the joy and vitality that menopause seems to have hidden away.

In Part 1, "Menopause 101," we'll dive into the basics, demystifying what's happening in your body and why. You'll gain a deeper understanding of this phase of life, empowering you to navigate it with confidence.

In Part 2, "Side Effects and Symptoms," tackles the nitty-gritty. From managing early menopause to handling mood swings, sexual changes, hair woes, sleep disruptions, memory challenges, and the often-frustrating battle with weight gain, each chapter is a guide tailored to your unique experiences.

In Part 3, "Natural Remedies and Resources," we'll explore holistic approaches. From alternative medicine to supplements and finding support, you'll discover a treasure trove of resources to support your journey towards wellness.

Before this information was available, finding relief from menopausal symptoms could feel like searching for a needle in a haystack. But with the insights and strategies shared in this book, you'll feel empowered, informed, and equipped to navigate this phase with grace and resilience.

So, if you've ever felt alone on your menopausal journey, wondering if there's a better way forward, rest assured, this is the right book for you.

Get ready to turn the page to Chapter 1, where we'll embark on your guide to menopause, unraveling the mysteries and empowering you to reclaim your vitality.

Let's begin this transformative journey together.

PART I
MENOPAUSE 101

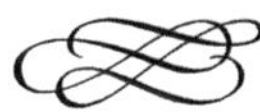

PART I
MENOPAUSE 101

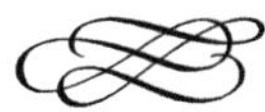

YOUR GUIDE TO MENOPAUSE

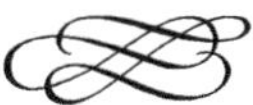

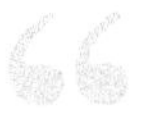

> *Menopause is like autumn leaves falling; it's a natural shedding of the old to make way for the new.*
>
> — PATRICIA AKINS

Most girls typically start menstruating around the age of 12, continuing with monthly cycles until they reach menopause. By the time women enter this phase of life, they have experienced approximately 450 menstrual periods (Coppa, n.d.). In the United States alone, more than a million women go through menopause annually. Despite its prevalence, there is still limited understanding of the impact of menopause on women's health. Researchers are actively investigating the causes of menopausal symptoms to support women of diverse racial and ethnic backgrounds in leading healthier lives throughout the menopausal transition and beyond (*Research Explores the Impact of Menopause on Women's Health and Aging*, 2022).

WHAT IS MENOPAUSE?

Menopause is a natural biological process that marks the end of your reproductive years. It typically occurs between the ages of 45 and 55, with the average age being around 51. However, the timing can vary widely among individuals. It is a significant milestone in a woman's life, signaling the end of menstrual periods and the end of fertility.

Symptoms

Symptoms can vary in severity and duration among women. Common symptoms include:

- Changes in libido: Decreased sex drive or changes in sexual response.
- Changes in skin and hair: Dry skin, hair thinning, and changes in hair texture.
- Hot flashes: Sudden feelings of intense heat, often accompanied by sweating and flushed skin.
- Memory lapses: Difficulty concentrating, brain fog, and forgetfulness.
- Mood swings: Emotional fluctuations, including irritability, feelings of anxiety, and depression.
- Night sweats: Hot flashes that happen when asleep, leading to disrupted sleep patterns.
- Sleep disturbances: Difficulty falling or staying asleep, often due to night sweats.
- Urinary changes: Increased frequency of urination or urinary incontinence.
- Vaginal dryness: Reduced vaginal lubrication, leading to discomfort or pain during intercourse.

Impact on Health and Well-Being

The decrease in estrogen levels can lead to several health concerns, including:

- Bone density loss: Reduced estrogen levels increase the risk of osteoporosis.
- Emotional health: Menopausal symptoms, combined with hormonal changes, can impact emotional well-being, contributing to mood swings, anxiety, and depression for some of us.
- Heart health: Estrogen plays a role in maintaining heart health, so the decline in estrogen levels can contribute to an increased risk of heart disease.
- Weight changes: Hormonal fluctuations can affect metabolism and body composition, leading to weight gain, particularly around the abdomen.

WHAT'S THE POINT?

Menopause has intrigued scientists for years. While several theories have been proposed to explain why it happens, it's important to note that the exact cause remains unclear, and these theories are the current hypotheses:

THE GRANDMOTHER HYPOTHESIS

It suggests that menopause evolved as a result of the benefits that older women could provide to their families and communities. These benefits include caregiving, sharing knowledge and resources, and helping to raise grandchildren. The theory implies that menopause may have evolved as a way to promote the survival and well-being of offspring and extended family members. Keep in mind that while this hypothesis offers a compelling explanation, it is still a hypothesis and not definitively proven (Powledge, 2008).

THE MOTHER HYPOTHESIS

It proposes that menopause occurs because of the increased risk of reproductive complications, like miscarriages and chromosomal abnormalities, as women age. By ending fertility at a certain age, women reduce the likelihood of passing on genetic defects or experiencing pregnancy-related health risks. Like the grandmother hypothesis, it provides a plausible explanation for menopause but is not conclusively proven (Powledge, 2008).

TRAIT EVOLVED THROUGH NATURAL SELECTION

Though the precise mechanisms are still up for debate, some experts say menopause may have emerged through natural selection. They speculate that terminating reproductive capacity at a specific age may have provided prehistoric populations with survival advantages, like lowering the likelihood of birthing difficulties or raising overall survival rates. The exact evolutionary forces that gave rise to menopause, however, are complicated and not very well understood (Almansa, 2022).

REDUCED RISK OF MISCARRIAGES AS WOMEN AGE—SURVIVAL BENEFIT

Another theory proposes that menopause evolved to reduce the risk of miscarriages and pregnancy-related complications as women age.

By ending fertility at a certain point, women may have been able to avoid the potential risks and health consequences associated with geriatric pregnancies, leading to improved overall survival rates for both mothers and babies. This theory underscores the potential survival benefits associated with menopause but is part of the broader discussion surrounding the evolutionary origins of this phenomenon.

While these hypotheses provide intriguing explanations for the evolution of menopause, it's important to remember that the exact cause is still unknown. These theories represent the ongoing efforts to understand this complex biological process and its implications for human evolution and reproductive health.

HOW CAN YOU TELL IF IT IS MENOPAUSE

- Increased risk of health conditions: Menopause is associated with an increased risk of osteoporosis, heart disease, and metabolic changes.
- Hot Flushes/Night Sweats: Hot flushes, or hot flashes, are spontaneous feelings of intense heat, often accompanied by sweating and flushed skin. Night sweats are hot flashes that happen when you sleep, leading to disjointed sleep.
- Menstrual Cycle Changes: Menstrual changes are one of the hallmark signs of approaching menopause. This includes irregular periods, changes in flow, and, eventually, the ending of periods.
- Mood Changes: Menopause can be accompanied by mood swings, including irritability, anxiety, and depression. Hormonal changes and the psychological impact of menopause may contribute to these mood changes.
- Muscle or Joint Pain: Muscle and joint pain can occur, leading to discomfort and reduced mobility.
- Physical Changes: Physical changes include changes in skin and hair texture, weight gain, and changes in body composition.
- Problems Sleeping: Menopausal women often experience sleep disturbances, including difficulty falling asleep or staying asleep.
- Trouble Focusing and Learning: Some women experience cognitive changes, like trouble focusing, memory lapses, and difficulty taking in new information. Concentration problems are widespread and may be directly related to the effects of low estrogen on brain function.

- Vaginal and Urinary Symptoms: Vaginal symptoms like dryness, itching, and discomfort during intercourse are common during menopause due to reduced estrogen levels. Urinary symptoms include increased frequency, urinary incontinence, or urinary tract infections.

This is just an overview of the range of symptoms that women may experience. Individual experiences can vary, and some women may experience only a few symptoms, while others may experience a combination of several. Understanding these symptoms can help us recognize and manage the challenges associated with menopause.

PHASES OF MENOPAUSE

Phase 1—Perimenopause

This phase begins several years before menopause, usually in your late 40s, but can start earlier for some. During perimenopause, hormone levels fluctuate a lot, leading to irregular menstrual cycles, changes in flow, and symptoms like hot flashes, night sweats, mood swings, and vaginal dryness.

Phase 2—Menopause

Menopause is officially declared after 12 consecutive months without a period. At this stage, the ovaries stop releasing eggs, and estrogen and progesterone production decreases. This shift causes the hallmark symptoms like hot flashes, night sweats, sleep disturbances, mood changes, and vaginal dryness.

Phase 3—Post-Menopause

Post-menopause refers to the years following menopause. During this phase, uncomfortable symptoms like hot flashes start to diminish, but other health concerns related to hormonal changes, like bone density loss (osteoporosis) and the risk of heart disease, become more prominent.

We've explored the journey of menopause. We delved into its phases, each with its unique challenges and experiences. Menopause brings with it a variety of symptoms, from hot flashes and sleep disturbances to mood swings and changes in libido, impacting both physical and emotional well-being.

Understanding the symptoms and implications of menopause helps us stay on top of our health and well-being. By recognizing and addressing these changes, we can navigate this phase with greater ease and maintain our overall health. Next, we will delve deeper into strategies and approaches to support you during this transitional period.

MANAGING EARLY MENOPAUSE

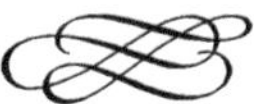

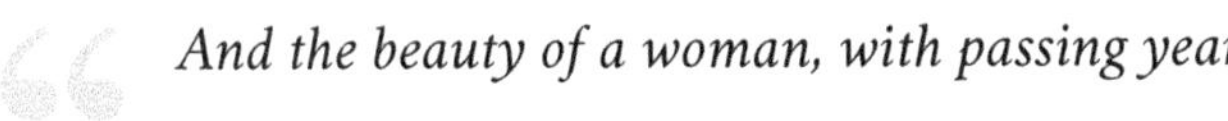

And the beauty of a woman, with passing years only grows!

— AUDREY HEPBURN

WHAT IS EARLY MENOPAUSE?

Approximately five percent of women experience early menopause, while premature menopause affects about one percent of women. In rare cases, menopause can occur in a woman's 20s, affecting roughly 0.1% of women (*Premature and Early Menopause: Causes, Diagnosis, and Treatment*, 2022). Early menopause typically happens before age 45, with premature menopause occurring before age 40. Menopause can start as early as one's 20s, but it's uncommon before 30 and is considered premature menopause.

Early menopause refers to the complete stopping of menstrual periods before the age of 45. Menopause typically occurs between the ages of 45 and 55. When this transition happens earlier, it is categorized as either early menopause or premature menopause, depending on the age at which it occurs.

Early Menopause vs. Premature Menopause

The distinction between the two is primarily based on age:

Early menopause: Occurs when a woman experiences menopause between the ages of 40 and 45. It affects approximately five percent of women.

Premature menopause: Occurs when menopause happens before the age of 40. It's less common, affecting about one percent of women. It is sometimes referred to as premature ovarian insufficiency (POI).

Both conditions involve the decline of ovarian function earlier than the average age for menopause. The terminology helps differentiate the timing and potentially different underlying causes and implications.

Premature Menopause vs. Premature Ovarian Failure

While premature menopause and premature ovarian failure might seem similar, they are two different conditions:

- Premature menopause: This is a permanent end to menstruation and the ability to conceive naturally. The ovaries stop releasing eggs and producing estrogen and progesterone (Arvind, 2023).
- Premature ovarian failure (POF): Also known as primary ovarian insufficiency (POI), does not always mean a permanent end to menstruation. Women with POF may still have irregular periods and could potentially conceive because the ovaries might still occasionally release eggs. POF involves reduced ovarian function before the age of 40, but it is not as absolute as premature menopause.

Earliest Age for Menopause

The earliest age at which menopause can occur naturally is in a woman's 20s or 30s, but this is extremely rare. The average age for natural menopause is around 51, but factors like genetics, medical treatments, and health conditions can influence the timing.

CAUSES OF EARLY MENOPAUSE

- Genetics: Family history plays a huge role. If one's mother or sister experienced early menopause, she is more likely to experience it as well.
- Autoimmune Diseases: Conditions like thyroid disease or rheumatoid arthritis can cause the immune system to attack the ovaries, leading to early menopause.
- Medical Treatments: Chemotherapy and radiation therapy can damage the ovaries and lead to early menopause. Also, surgical removal of the ovaries (oophorectomy) induces immediate menopause.
- Infections: Some viral infections can damage the ovaries and lead to premature ovarian failure.
- Lifestyle Factors: Smoking, for instance, has been linked to an earlier onset of menopause.

Implications of Early Menopause

- Health Risks: Early or premature menopause puts one at a higher risk for health conditions like osteoporosis and cardiovascular disease because of the prolonged period of low estrogen levels.
- Fertility Concerns: Early and premature menopause can impact a woman's ability to conceive naturally, often leading to considerations of fertility preservation or other family planning methods.

- Emotional and Psychological Impact: The unexpected and early transition into menopause can cause emotional distress, anxiety, and depression because of the abrupt end of fertility and the onset of menopausal symptoms at a younger age.

THE CAUSES OF PREMATURE MENOPAUSE

Premature menopause, while hormonally similar to natural menopause, occurs at a much younger age. The ovaries stop producing estrogen, and ovulation stops. However, there are instances where the ovaries might sporadically release an egg, enabling conception as thousands of eggs remain within the ovaries. It's important to note that premature menopause does not signify premature aging; rather, it indicates a malfunction in ovarian function. Several factors can lead to it:

- Family History: Women with a family history of early or premature menopause are more likely to experience it themselves. Genetics plays a role in determining the onset of menopause.
- Smoking: Smoking can accelerate the onset of menopause by up to two years compared to non-smokers. Smoking is also associated with more severe menopausal symptoms.
- Surgical Removal of the Uterus (Hysterectomy): Women who undergo a hysterectomy can retain their ovaries, which will continue to produce hormones. But they cannot conceive, and their periods stop; they do not experience immediate menopause. Natural menopause may occur a few years earlier than expected, though.
- Surgical Removal of the Ovaries (Bilateral Oophorectomy): The removal of both ovaries leads to the onset of immediate menopause. Hormone levels drop sharply, ending periods and often resulting in severe menopausal symptoms like hot flashes and decreased libido.

- Cancer Therapies: Chemotherapy and pelvic radiation can damage the ovaries, leading to a temporary or permanent stop of menstruation. These treatments can impair fertility. The risk of induced menopause varies, with younger women being less likely to experience menopause from these therapies.
- Autoimmune Diseases: Rheumatoid arthritis and thyroid disorders can cause the immune system to attack the ovaries, hindering hormone production and leading to premature menopause.
- HIV and AIDS: Women with poorly managed HIV may experience early menopause. HIV-positive women also often have more intense hot flashes compared to non-HIV-infected women.
- Chromosomal Abnormalities: Genetic conditions like Turner's syndrome, where there is a missing or incomplete X chromosome, can result in early menopause. These women often have irregular menstrual cycles and may have underdeveloped ovaries.
- Chronic Fatigue Syndrome or Myalgic encephalomyelitis/chronic fatigue syndrome (ME/CFS): Women with ME/CFS often experience symptoms like extreme fatigue, muscle and joint pain, headaches, memory issues, and unsatisfying sleep. Research indicates that these women are more likely to undergo early or premature menopause.

Understanding the distinctions between early menopause, premature menopause, and premature ovarian failure helps you know when to seek appropriate care and support. Early intervention and management can help mitigate health risks and improve the quality of life.

SURGICAL MENOPAUSE

Surgical menopause occurs as a direct consequence of a medical procedure rather than the natural aging process. It usually follows an oophorectomy, which is the surgical removal of the ovaries. Since the ovaries are the body's main source of estrogen production, their removal leads to an immediate onset of menopause, irrespective of age. This abrupt change can trigger a range of menopausal symptoms almost instantly.

An oophorectomy can be performed on its own or in conjunction with a hysterectomy, a procedure where the uterus is removed. While a hysterectomy alone stops one's periods, it does not induce menopause unless the ovaries are also taken out. This combination of surgeries is sometimes chosen to reduce the risk of chronic illnesses, like certain types of cancer.

When both ovaries are removed, the body loses its primary source of estrogen, leading to a sudden and significant drop in hormone levels. This can cause more severe menopausal symptoms compared to natural menopause, where hormonal changes occur more gradually. The decision to undergo the procedures is often based on medical conditions like ovarian cancer, severe endometriosis, or preventive measures for those with a high risk of certain cancers.

Understanding the implications of surgical menopause is crucial for managing the associated health and emotional challenges effectively.

The duration of these symptoms varies greatly from one woman to another. While some may see them resolve on their own over time, others might experience prolonged issues. If these symptoms disrupt your daily life, it's good to consult with your healthcare provider. They can assess your situation and refer you to specialists if need be, ensuring that you receive the support and treatment you need to manage your symptoms effectively.

Thinking About Your Long-Term Health

Following surgical menopause, your doctor will offer guidance on how you can maintain your long-term health. This advice will focus on keeping your heart healthy and preventing osteoporosis, a condition characterized by weak, brittle bones. Early menopause can increase the risk of osteoporosis, which in turn raises the likelihood of fractures. To assess your bone strength and density, you should undergo a DEXA scan (Dual-Energy X-ray Absorptiometry). The scan will help predict your future risk of fractures. Here are some steps you can take to protect your long-term health:

- Hormone Replacement Therapy: HRT can help prevent bone density loss and reduce the risk of heart disease. Discuss with your healthcare team whether it is suitable for you, given your medical history and health status.
- A Calcium-Rich Diet: A balanced diet rich in calcium is important. Aim for approximately 700 mg of calcium per day. Good sources include dairy products, sardines, chocolate, almonds, and oranges.
- Regular Exercise: Engage in regular, moderate exercise. This should include both aerobic activities (to increase your heart rate) and weight-bearing exercises (supporting your body weight through standing or using your arms and hands).
- Lifestyle Adjustments: Avoid smoking, drink alcohol in moderation, and maintain a healthy weight.

Discuss your options thoroughly with your healthcare provider to make informed decisions about your health post-surgery.

Potential Benefits of Surgical Menopause

For some women, surgical menopause through ovarian removal can be life-saving. Estrogen can fuel certain types of cancers, leading to their development at a younger age in some women. Those with a family history of breast or ovarian cancer are particularly vulnerable because of potential genetic factors that prevent tumor growth inhibition. In such cases, an oophorectomy can serve as a preventive measure to significantly reduce the risk of developing these cancers.

Also, surgical menopause can alleviate the discomfort associated with endometriosis, a condition where uterine tissue grows outside the uterus, causing severe pelvic pain and potentially damaging the lymph nodes, fallopian tubes, or ovaries. An oophorectomy can reduce the pain, but women with this condition typically are not candidates for HRT.

WHY OOPHORECTOMIES ARE PERFORMED

An oophorectomy is generally performed as a preventive measure against illness. Women with a significant family history of cancer may be advised by their doctors to remove one or both ovaries to lower the risk of tumors affecting their reproductive system. In some cases, uterine removal may also be necessary.

Other reasons for opting for ovarian removal include the management of endometriosis symptoms and chronic pelvic pain. While there are successful cases where oophorectomy alleviates pain, it is not always effective. Consequently, removing healthy ovaries to treat other pelvic conditions is generally not recommended.

Women might also choose surgical menopause and ovarian removal for other health reasons, like:

Ovarian torsion: Twisted ovaries that affect blood flow.

Recurrent ovarian cysts: Persistent cysts that cause significant pain and discomfort.

Benign ovarian tumors: Non-cancerous tumors that may still cause health issues.

While surgical menopause through oophorectomy can offer significant health benefits and preventive measures for certain women, it is important to weigh the risks and consult with a healthcare provider to make the best-informed decision.

ARE PREMATURE MENOPAUSE AND MENOPAUSE SYMPTOMS THE SAME?

It is important to understand the distinction between premature menopause and normal menopause. Despite the difference in timing, the symptoms of premature menopause and regular menopause can be quite similar. However, there are nuances in intensity and impact, especially if the onset of menopause is because of surgical or medical interventions like cancer treatments.

While the symptoms are similar, the onset of premature menopause, particularly when caused by surgical procedures like oophorectomy or cancer treatments, can lead to more intense and sudden symptoms. This is because the body has less time to gradually adjust to the decrease in hormone levels.

Diagnosing Premature Menopause

Diagnosing premature menopause involves several steps to ensure accurate identification and appropriate management. If a woman under 45 experiences irregular periods or if her periods stop for more than three months, she needs to consult a healthcare provider. The diagnosis process normally includes:

- Medical and Family History: The doctor will inquire about one's medical history, family history of menopause, and any symptoms experienced.
- Physical Examination: A thorough physical exam to check for signs of hormonal changes.

- Blood Tests: These tests measure hormone levels, including follicle-stimulating hormone (FSH) and estradiol, to determine if the ovaries are functioning properly.
- Other Tests: Depending on the patient's history and symptoms, additional tests like thyroid function tests, pelvic ultrasound, or genetic testing may be conducted to rule out other causes.

When to Seek Medical Advice

Seek medical advice if you are under the age of 45 and experiencing the following:

- Irregular Periods: If your cycle becomes irregular or stops for more than three months, see your doctor.
- Menopausal Symptoms: Experiencing symptoms commonly associated with menopause should prompt a consultation with your doctor.

During the consultation, your doctor may ask about:

- Menstrual History: Details about your cycle patterns, including any changes or irregularities.
- Symptoms: A description of the symptoms you are experiencing, their frequency, and their impact on your daily life.
- Lifestyle Factors: Information about your diet, exercise habits, stress levels, and any use of tobacco, alcohol, or drugs.
- Family History: Whether there is a history of premature menopause or related conditions in your family.

Understanding early menopause is crucial for women who experience this transition prematurely. Early menopause presents unique challenges that can significantly impact physical, emotional, and reproductive health. The distinction between early and premature menopause highlights the importance of recognizing the timing and potential causes, like genetics, medical treatments, autoimmune diseases, and lifestyle factors. Awareness and early intervention can help mitigate health risks, like osteoporosis and cardiovascular disease, and provide strategies for managing symptoms effectively. For those facing this early transition, seeking appropriate medical care and support is essential in navigating the complexities of early menopause and maintaining overall well-being. Now that we know more about what menopause is and what we can expect, we can take a more in-depth look at symptoms and side effects.

PART II
SIDE EFFECTS AND SYMPTOMS

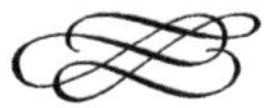

SIDE EFFECTS AND SYMPTOMS

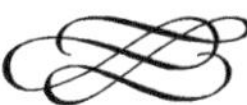

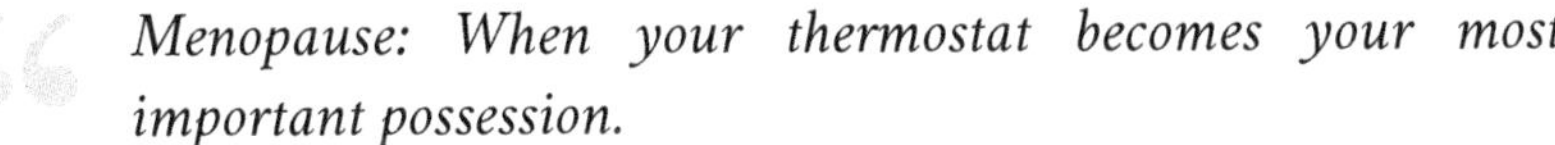

> *Menopause: When your thermostat becomes your most important possession.*
>
> — ANONYMOUS

Over 90% of postmenopausal women never received instruction about menopause in school, and over 60% of them didn't begin researching the topic until after their symptoms had begun. In May 2021, 829 postmenopausal women participated in an online survey that was used to gather data for the study. The menopause was judged to be uninformed by 49% of participants, and 62.7% of women reported that it was either tough or extremely difficult (UCL, 2023).

MONUMENTAL MELTDOWNS

Meet Lauren, a 45-year-old woman navigating the tumultuous waters of perimenopause. She had always been known for her calm and composed demeanor. As a mother of two and a successful professional, she prided herself on her ability to handle stress. However, as she entered perimenopause, she found herself facing unexpected and overwhelming emotional surges that left her feeling out of control.

The Emotional Rollercoaster

As she transitioned into menopause, she began experiencing severe hormonal fluctuations that drastically altered her emotional landscape. She noticed herself becoming irritable over the smallest things, something completely out of character for her. She would swing from moments of intense anger to deep sadness, often without any apparent reason. These emotional changes were not only confusing but also frightening for her because she felt like she was losing control over her own emotions.

Extreme Rage Incident

One particular incident stands out in Lauren's mind as a stark example of how menopause affected her emotionally. It was a Saturday afternoon, and she was at home with her family. Her son had accidentally spilled a glass of juice on the freshly cleaned kitchen floor. Ordinarily, she would have handled the situation with a simple sigh and a reminder to be more careful. But on that day, she felt an overwhelming surge of rage. Her heart raced, her face flushed, and she could feel her blood pressure skyrocketing. Before she knew it, she was yelling at her son, her voice filled with anger and frustration.

Her husband and son were taken aback by her outburst. Her son apologized repeatedly, tears welling up in his eyes, but she found it difficult to calm down. The rational part of her knew that her reaction was over the top, but she felt powerless to control the anger that was boiling inside her. After the incident, she retreated to her bedroom, filled with guilt and confusion. She couldn't understand why she had reacted so strongly to something so minor.

Lauren's experience with extreme rage was a wake-up call. She realized that she needed help to manage these emotional changes. She began researching and learning more about the hormonal fluctuations that occur at this stage of life. She discovered that she was not alone in her experiences. Many women going through menopause reported similar episodes of intense anger and mood swings.

Determined to regain control over her emotions, she sought the guidance of a healthcare professional. She learned some strategies to manage her symptoms, including lifestyle changes, stress management techniques, and hormone replacement therapy. She also joined a support group for women experiencing menopause, where she could share her experiences and hear from others who were going through similar challenges.

Through a combination of medical intervention, support from loved ones, and personal effort, Lauren gradually began to feel more like herself. She learned to recognize the early signs of an impending emotional surge and developed techniques to manage her reactions. While the journey was not easy, she emerged stronger and more self-aware, equipped with the tools to navigate the rest of her menopausal transition with greater ease.

Lauren's story is a powerful reminder of the profound impact menopause can have on your emotional well-being. The hormonal surges associated with this stage of life can lead to intense and often uncontrollable emotional responses. Understanding that these reactions are a natural part of the process and seeking appropriate support can make a big difference. Lauren's journey highlights the importance of acknowledging these changes, seeking help, and finding strategies to manage the emotional challenges of menopause.

WHY AM I ALWAYS SO ANGRY?

Before menopause, during the perimenopause phase, all of the usual symptoms will manifest. Your body may react to changes in your reproductive hormone levels with mood swings, sleep disturbances, and hot flashes. Occasionally, these mood swings manifest as abrupt, strong emotions like panic, anxiety, or rage. Menopausal-related variables may contribute to feelings of rage. Unstable moods can be exacerbated by the reality of aging and transitioning into a new stage of life, as well as the stress that occasionally results from sleep deprivation and hot flashes. Keep in mind that although your body is changing, these feelings are not your fault. There's a chemical reaction happening here. Menopause anger is challenging to categorize as frequent or uncommon because menopause affects women differently. Although hormonal fluctuations might have a big impact on your mood, this doesn't imply you'll always be unable to manage how you feel.

Here is why mood swings during this incredible phase in our life: Most of a woman's reproductive processes are controlled by the hormone estrogen. The ovaries decrease their estrogen production as you get closer to menopause. The amount of serotonin generated in your brain is likewise regulated by estrogen. The neurotransmitter serotonin aids with mood regulation. Reduced estrogen production is accompanied by decreased serotonin production. How confident and positive you feel may directly be affected by this. The secret to regaining control over your mood is hormone balance. It may be possible to naturally balance your hormones by engaging in a variety of activities and making lifestyle adjustments.

OTHER EMOTIONS THAT ARE HEIGHTENED

Dealing with something you have some comprehension of makes things easier, as is the case with most things in life. Keeping this in mind, have a look at a few emotional symptoms brought on by an imbalance in the hormones that typically control mood and emotions:

- absence of motivation
- anxiety and nervousness
- fatigue, which might also result from sleep deprivation
- heightened irritability or a complete lack of patience

- hostility
- inability to focus and forgetfulness
- intolerance
- sadness, hopelessness, and depressive feelings
- feelings of heightened tension or stress

These mood swings can occur frequently, be severe, and start quickly. Other than the feeling that something is off, some of the feelings are inexplicable.

CHANNELING YOUR EMOTIONS

Expressing our emotions, whether positive or negative, is necessary in the moments when we need an outlet. Our lives are busy, so it's easy to overlook giving emotions the time they deserve for processing. It's tempting to dismiss feelings like annoyance, anger, or self-doubt as hormonal, but this approach rarely benefits us or our relationships. The good news is that there are ways to channel these emotions, turning negativity into positivity.

- Release: Low serotonin levels may not always cause anger, but they can make it harder to control, suppress, or hide anger. There are times when expressing anger, directed appropriately and constructively, is valid and necessary. Imagine the relief of finally sharing the truths you've kept bottled up for so long, embracing openness, honesty, and authenticity like never before.
- Let go of guilt: It's normal to lose your composure occasionally, especially during this phase of life. Cut yourself some slack. Communicate your struggles openly with loved ones and try to minimize any unintended consequences. Be ready to apologize when necessary, acknowledge your mistakes, and move forward.
- Harness the energy: Use the intensity of anger as a catalyst for finding solutions. With decades of life experience behind you,

leverage your skills in arguing, resilience, and wisdom to address challenges. Take deep breaths to center yourself before expressing your thoughts.

- Self-care: While vigorous exercise might not be ideal when angry, physical activity can boost your mood and calmness. A brisk walk or a session with a punching bag can ground you when you feel overwhelmed. Prioritize nutrition to support hormonal balance, especially if you're embracing honesty and openness fully.
- Explore new avenues: Direct your adrenaline or energy into productive things. Try a new hobby, start journaling, or cook a dish that mirrors your passionate feelings. Positively channeling this energy can lead to a sense of accomplishment and fulfillment.

Mood swings, anxiety, and bursts of anger are common, but they need not define your journey. Reclaiming emotional control and embracing this new phase can be aided by medical guidance, natural remedies, and personal outlets tailored to your needs.

KNOWING WHAT DEPRESSION LOOKS LIKE

In theory, menopause is a single day that happens 12 months following your last menstrual cycle. You are then classified as post-menopausal. Prior to that, you go through perimenopause, a time when your reproductive hormones are changing and may increase your risk of developing severe depression.

Changes in hormone levels: Your menstrual cycle might grow longer, shorter, heavier, lighter, more frequent, or closer together during this period. Reduced hormone levels might cause mood fluctuations that make it harder for you to handle situations you would otherwise be able to handle. Some people experience depressive episodes as a result of these hormone drops, particularly those who have already had severe depression.

Issues with sleep: Sleeplessness is due, in part, to hot flashes that occur at night. A lack of sleep can increase your risk of developing depression by up to ten times.

Changes in life: Aside from volatile hormones, this may be a stressful time in life due to things like aging parents, pressure from work, health issues, and children moving out. These outside influences have the potential to worsen mood swings and either cause or exacerbate depression.

Depression is a mood disorder that impairs one's ability to feel, think, and carry out everyday tasks. It is characterized by enduring emotions of melancholy or disinterest. Major (clinical) depression and chronic depressive disorder (dysthymia) are the two most prevalent types. Sadness, loss of interest in activities you used to like, impatience, exhaustion, and thoughts of worthlessness, despair, and pessimism, coupled with physical symptoms, are common signs of depression.

Hormonal changes, pre-existing depression vulnerabilities, and other stresses are some of the variables that can cause depressive symptoms to manifest during perimenopause and menopause. Hormonal changes that occur throughout other stages of your reproductive life, like the postpartum phase, are also linked to a rise in symptoms of depression and mood disorders. Nevertheless, there is no proof that depression is brought on by menopause. Make sure to visit your physician or a mental health professional if your symptoms are severe or significantly affecting your life on a regular basis.

In order to assess where you are in the menopausal transition and suggest the next steps for potentially treating menopausal symptoms, your doctor might conduct an examination. However, seeing a mental health professional for evaluation is the next step if your depression symptoms are severe or if you've already received a diagnosis. Also, keep in mind that if you struggle to cope with your thoughts, it is essential to seek help as soon as possible.

WHAT CAN HELP

Once diagnosed, a combination of psychotherapy and antidepressants may be used to treat your depression. Serotonin and norepinephrine reuptake inhibitors (SNRIs) or selective serotonin reuptake inhibitors (SSRIs) may be recommended by doctors for menopause-related mood disorders. Depressive symptoms may be lessened by these drugs by upping neurotransmitter levels. Also, they could improve one's condition sufficiently for psychotherapy to start. Finding the causes of depression can be made easier with the use of psychotherapy. An individual seeking therapy can better understand and control their feelings. According to a 2018 study (West, 2021), perimenopausal depression has not been given Food and Drug Administration (FDA) approval for the use of estrogen treatment. Hot flashes, sleep issues, and other symptoms that could impact your mood, however, might be lessened with this therapy.

Complimentary Therapy

Complementary therapy, especially for perimenopausal depression, is not well-researched. Nonetheless, the following actions can be taken to assist with menopausal symptoms, depression, or both:

- Exercise on a regular basis.
- Limiting alcohol and caffeine intake, especially for people who have trouble sleeping.
- Doing yoga or tai chi can assist with stress reduction and sleep.
- Entering into hypnosis, which can aid with hot flash frequency from a reliable source.

Living a healthy lifestyle is a great way to help in relieving symptoms. Your health is very important, so it is imperative that you take care of yourself in the best way possible.

USING MINDFULNESS MEDITATION

A new study from the Mayo Clinic suggests that women who practice mindfulness may have fewer menopausal symptoms. Researchers found that menopausal women who struggle with anger, anxiety, and sadness may benefit most from practicing mindfulness (Kehren, 2019). Being mindful means paying attention to the here and now and objectively examining all your thoughts and feelings.

Yoga, tai chi, and qigong are just a few disciplines and practices that can cultivate mindfulness. However, the majority of the literature has concentrated on mindfulness, which is developed through mindfulness meditation, which is a self-regulation practice that trains attention and awareness to bring mental processes under greater voluntary control and thereby foster general mental development and well-being, as well as specific capacities like calmness, clarity, and concentration.

More Benefits of Mindfulness Meditation

Through working memory gains, mindfulness meditation increases metacognitive awareness, reduces rumination by disengaging from perseverative cognitive activity, and improves attention skills. Effective emotion regulation techniques are subsequently influenced by these cognitive advances. Here are some of the benefits:

Reduced rumination: Generalized rumination becomes less self-perpetuating and uncontrolled when you practice mindfulness. Metacognition, or understanding of your own mental process, reduces self-critical rumination. Meditation strengthens this kind of awareness.

Reduced stress: Consider trying meditation if stress is making you feel tense, worried, and anxious. Even a short meditation session might help you regain your composure and inner serenity.

Boosted working memory: Working memory improvements seem to be yet another advantage of mindfulness. Meditation appears to be negatively correlated with negative effects and directly connected to good effects.

Focus: Enhancing your working memory, increasing your attention span, and decreasing mind-wandering are some of the ways that mindfulness and meditation help you become more focused. The capacity to maintain focus on an activity or task for an extended amount of time is known as attention span.

Reduced emotional reactivity: In the brain regions responsible for memory, learning, empathy, and emotional regulation, mindfulness can lead to an increase in gray matter. It gives you time to become more aware of your feelings, thoughts, and wants by allowing you to slow down. Raising your self-compassion and lowering your emotional reactivity can help you better control your emotions.

More cognitive flexibility: Being mindful makes it easier to see things from several angles, adjust our strategy to suit the circumstances, and achieve the greatest outcome. In other words, it's important to give each assignment or task your full attention and to do it as well as possible.

Relationship satisfaction: Healthy relationships are facilitated by mindfulness, which also improves acceptance, emotion control, and the ability to modify yourself for the betterment of your relationships. Being more conscious and welcoming, as well as purposeful in your interactions with your family and friends, are all possible with mindfulness.

How to Use Mindfulness

Establishing a practice time limit before starting can help prevent fixation on giving up. Start with a short period, gradually increasing to an hour or 45 minutes. You are welcome to use a timer to track the time you spend. Despite busy schedules, taking action is better than doing nothing. Here is how to do it:

1. Have a seat. Choose a position where you can sit with stability and support without leaning forward or sagging, whether it's a chair, a meditation cushion, or a bench of some sort.
2. Take note of your leg movements. Spread your legs apart comfortably in front of you as if you're sitting on a floor cushion. If you are currently practicing sitting yoga poses, feel free to continue. It's better if your feet are flat on the ground when seated on a chair.
3. Make your upper body straight, but avoid becoming rigid. The spine has a natural curvature. Give it permission to form. On top of your vertebrae, your head and shoulders can rest comfortably.
4. Hold your upper arms in a position parallel to your upper torso. After this, let your hands land on your legs. Your hands will land in the proper place if you keep your upper arms at your sides. You'll stoop if you move ahead too much. It will stiffen if you look too far back. You're fine-tuning the muscles in your body so they're neither too tight nor too loose.
5. Lower your chin a bit and softly direct your attention downward. You can open your eyes wider. When meditating, it's not necessary to close your eyes; however, you can if you feel the need to. You can just let what's in front of your eyes exist without giving it much attention.
6. Spend a few moments there. Unwind. Focus on your breathing or the feelings that are happening within your body.
7. Feel your breath as it comes in and goes out, or as some people say, "follow" it. In certain variations of this exercise, the emphasis is mostly on the exhale, while the inhale is just met with a broad pause. In either case, focus on the physical aspects of breathing, like the air passing through your mouth or nose, your abdomen rising and falling, or the sensations in

your chest. Choose your concentration point, and mentally record *breathing in* and *breathing out* with each breath.

8. Your focus will inevitably go from your breath and go elsewhere. Remain calm. Thinking does not need to be restricted or eliminated. Simply, gently bring your focus back to breathing when you eventually notice that your mind is straying—this might take a few seconds, a minute, or five minutes.
9. To avoid making any bodily changes, like shifting your body or scratching an itch, practice stopping first. Make a conscious decision to change at any time, creating a gap between your experiences and your actions.
10. It's also common for your thoughts to wander. Practice watching without feeling the urge to respond, as opposed to struggling with or interacting with those thoughts as much. Just take a seat and focus. That's it, as difficult as it is to maintain. Return time and time again with no expectations or judgment.
11. When you're prepared, raise your head slightly and open your closed eyes. Look around you for a bit and listen to any noises. Take note of your current physical feelings. Take note of your feelings and thoughts. After a brief pause, choose how you want to spend the rest of the day.

And that is all. Although it's said that if something is extremely simple, that doesn't necessarily mean it is always easy to do. You just need to persevere. In the end, there will be a long-term impact. Making the daily commitment to sit, even for just five minutes, is important. The most crucial part of your meditation practice is actually sitting down to meditate because, at that very moment, you're telling yourself that you believe in self-care and transformation, and you're making it happen.

Mindfulness Body Scan

You've got an idea by now about the many advantages of mindfulness and meditation. But there are so many different forms of meditation that you might not know where to begin. You can increase your awareness of your physical feelings by using the body scan method. With this understanding, it may be easier to treat emotional and physical issues, resulting in increased physical and mental well-being. Here are steps you can try:

1. Make yourself comfortable: You can sit or lie in a posture that lets you effortlessly extend your limbs.
2. Concentrate: Shut your eyes and concentrate on your breathing. As you inhale and exhale, pay attention to how your breath fills and exits your lungs.
3. Decide where to begin: Anywhere on your head, left foot, right hand, or right foot would be a good place to start. As you maintain your deep, calm breathing, concentrate on that area. Next, go to a different area of your body and repeat the process.
4. Be mindful: Allow yourself to be aware of any unusual feelings like pain, stress, or discomfort.
5. Move slowly: Allocate a duration of 20 seconds to 1 minute to observe these feelings.
6. Acknowledge: As soon as you start to feel pain and discomfort, accept and stay with any feelings that arise. Take them in without passing judgment. Don't criticize yourself, for instance, if you're upset or annoyed. Take note of them, feel them, and let them go.
7. Breathe: Breathe continuously, visualizing the tension and agony fading with each breath.
8. Let go: Gradually shift your attention from that particular body part to the next one you want to concentrate on. For some, it helps to visualize releasing one body part with each exhale and moving on to the next with each inhale.

9. Proceed: Whether you move up one side and down the other or from top to bottom, make sure you continue the workout with your body in a manner that makes sense to you.
10. Take note of straying thoughts: Take notice of any moments when your mind strays while you keep scanning your body. Don't worry; this will probably happen more than once. You can refocus your thoughts, and you haven't failed; slowly pick up where you left off with your awareness.
11. Breathe and visualize: Let your awareness move across your body after you've finished scanning certain areas of it. Imagine this as a liquid pouring into a mold. Sit for a few seconds with this awareness of your entire body, taking slow, deep breaths and letting them out.
12. Come back: Return your concentration to your surroundings by letting it go gradually.

Remember that if you approach it with defined goals, you may get so preoccupied with accomplishing them that you find it difficult to pay attention to your physical feelings. You may become even more anxious than before you started meditating if you start to feel like it's not working. It's better to start with a single, straightforward objective: become more knowledgeable about what your body is telling you.

We have delved into the emotional turmoil one could experience during menopause, using Lauren's story as a focal point to highlight the intense emotional surges many of us could face, ranging from irritability to extreme anger and sadness. We've emphasized the lack of preparation and knowledge among women entering menopause, leading to challenges in managing these changes. Understanding that these reactions are a natural part of the process is important, prompting the need to seek professional guidance, join support groups, and implement lifestyle changes to regain emotional control. This sets the stage for exploring further how menopause impacts various aspects of life, including intimacy and sexual health, in the upcoming chapter on "The Sexual Side Effects."

THE SEXUAL SIDE EFFECTS

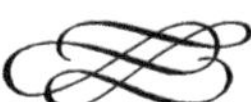

> *Menopause: When life gives you hot flashes, make margaritas.*
>
> — ANONYMOUS

Of the women going through menopause, 61% said that having a dry vagina makes having sex difficult, although 41% never use lubricants or other sex aids when having sex with a partner (*Bonafide Health*, 2021).

MENOPAUSE AND SEX

Understanding the changes in your body and knowing that they are normal can help you manage your symptoms and regain confidence in your sex life.

Common Sexual Issues Encountered During Menopause

Menopause can affect your sex life in various ways due to the hormonal shifts that influence physical and emotional well-being.

Vaginal Changes

Decreased estrogen levels can lead to vaginal dryness, thinning of the vaginal walls, and reduced elasticity. These changes tend to make intercourse uncomfortable or even painful. It's important to acknowledge that these symptoms are common and treatable aspects of menopause.

Bladder and Pelvic Floor Changes

Menopause can also bring about changes in the bladder and pelvic floor muscles. Weakened pelvic floor muscles can lead to urinary incontinence and reduced sexual satisfaction. Bladder sensitivity might increase, which would cause frequent urges to urinate, which would be disruptive during intimate moments.

Sexual Experience

The combination of vaginal changes, bladder issues, and reduced blood flow to the genital area alters the sexual experience. Women might find it harder to become aroused or reach orgasm. These changes can be frustrating, but they are manageable with the right strategies and treatments.

Low Sexual Desire

Most women experience a decrease in sexual desire during menopause. This can be due to hormonal changes, stress, fatigue, or feelings of depression and anxiety. Knowing that these feelings are common can lift some of the emotional burden associated with low libido.

Feeling Uncomfortable With Your Changing Body

Menopause often brings about changes in body shape and weight distribution, leading to low self-esteem and dissatisfaction with body image. Women may feel less attractive or desirable, which can negatively impact their sex life.

MANAGING SYMPTOMS AND REGAINING CONFIDENCE

Issues around sex during menopause are normal, but they don't have to be permanent or detrimental to your sex life. Here are some ways to manage symptoms and feel more confident:

1. Use moisturizers and lubricants: Over-the-counter vaginal moisturizers and lubricants can alleviate dryness and make intercourse more comfortable.
2. Pelvic floor exercises: Strengthening the pelvic floor muscles through exercises like Kegels can improve bladder control and enhance sexual satisfaction.
3. Open communication: Talking openly with your partner about your experiences and preferences can improve intimacy and reduce anxiety.
4. Professional help: A healthcare professional or a sex therapist can provide you with personalized strategies and treatments. Hormone replacement therapy (HRT) or vaginal estrogen creams can help with managing symptoms.
5. Body positivity: Embracing body changes and focusing on overall health can improve self-esteem. Practices like yoga, meditation, and mindfulness can also help you maintain a positive body image.
6. Explore new forms of intimacy: Expanding the definition of intimacy beyond intercourse can enhance your connection with your partner. Spending more time on foreplay, cuddling, and non-sexual physical touch can be deeply satisfying.

Actively managing your symptoms allows you to continue to enjoy a fulfilling and pleasurable sex life. Embracing this new phase with an open mind and seeking appropriate help can lead to a revitalized sense of intimacy and connection with your partner.

VAGINAL ATROPHY

Vaginal atrophy, or atrophic vaginitis, is a common yet under-discussed condition that significantly impacts a woman's quality of life, particularly during and after menopause. Understanding what it is, its symptoms, causes, and how to manage it can help women take proactive steps to maintain their vaginal health.

What Is Vaginal Atrophy?

It is the thinning, drying, and inflammation of the vaginal walls due to the decrease in estrogen levels. It is most common after menopause but can also occur during breastfeeding or as a side effect of treatments like chemotherapy or hormone therapy for breast cancer. The reduction in estrogen levels leads to a decrease in the natural lubrication and elasticity of the vaginal tissues, resulting in a range of uncomfortable symptoms (Sizensky & Berman, 2016).

Symptoms of Vaginal Atrophy—How It Feels

Symptoms can vary but include:

- Vaginal dryness: A persistent feeling of dryness in the vagina.
- Burning sensations: A burning sensation in the vaginal area, which can extend to the vulva.
- Itching: Itchiness around the vaginal and vulvar areas.
- Discomfort or pain during intercourse (Dyspareunia): Painful sexual intercourse because of reduced lubrication and elasticity.
- Vaginal discharge: A thin, watery discharge that can be clear or slightly yellow.
- Vaginal bleeding or spotting: Light bleeding or spotting, especially after intercourse.

- Urinary symptoms: Increased urinary frequency, urgency, burning during urination, and recurrent urinary tract infections (UTIs).

When to Consult a Healthcare Professional

It's important to consult a healthcare professional if you experience any of the symptoms above, especially if they interfere with your daily life or sexual activities. A doctor can provide a proper diagnosis and discuss the right treatment options. Early intervention can prevent symptoms from worsening and improve your quality of life.

CAUSES

The primary cause of vaginal atrophy is a decrease in estrogen levels. The decline can occur due to the following:

- Menopause: The most common cause.
- Breastfeeding: Temporary reduction in estrogen levels.
- Surgical removal of ovaries (Oophorectomy): It leads to a drop in estrogen.
- Cancer treatments: Chemotherapy or hormone therapy for breast cancer can affect estrogen levels.
- Medications: Some medications can reduce estrogen levels or block its effects.

RISK FACTORS

These are the factors that can increase the likelihood of developing vaginal atrophy:

- Smoking: Reduces blood circulation, leading to decreased oxygen supply to vaginal tissues.
- Lack of sexual activity: Regular sexual activity helps maintain healthy vaginal tissues by increasing blood flow.

- Not having given birth vaginally: Women who have not had vaginal deliveries may have an increased risk.
- Use of douches or perfumed soaps: They can irritate and dry out the vagina.

WHAT IS GSM?

Genitourinary syndrome (GSM) is a symptom of menopause because it produces symptoms related to both the bladder and the vagina. Signs and symptoms include:

- dryness in the vagina
- burning in the vagina
- discharge from the vagina
- vaginal itch
- burning while passing gas
- urgency with urination
- recurring urination
- urinary tract infections that come back frequently
- the inability to urinate
- light bleeding following sexual contact
- discomfort during sexual activity
- reduced lubrication in the vagina during intercourse; constriction and shortening of the vaginal canal

GSM is common in postmenopausal women, but very few of them seek help. Women sometimes decide to live with their symptoms instead of talking to their doctor about them because they feel ashamed. If you have any odd discharge, burning, pain, or unexplained spotting or bleeding, schedule an appointment with your doctor.

Doctors understand that anyone can deal with health issues, so the question to ask would be what the causes are. With GSM, there are a few to consider because there is a drop in estrogen levels. Causes include and may begin

- following menopause.
- the years preceding menopause or perimenopause.
- following surgical menopause.
- while nursing.
- when using drugs that might impact estrogen levels, like birth control tablets.
- after cancerous pelvic radiation treatment.
- after cancer chemotherapy.
- as an adverse consequence of hormone therapy for breast cancer.

Risk Factors

Smoking cigarettes has an adverse effect on blood circulation, which may reduce oxygen and blood flow to the vagina and other surrounding tissues. Also, smoking lessens the effects of estrogens that are naturally present in your body.

Absence of sexual activity: Engaging in sexual activity, whether with or without a partner, tightens your vaginal tissues and boosts blood flow.

Not a single vaginal delivery: Women who have never had a baby vaginally are more likely than those who have to deal with GSM symptoms (*Vaginal Atrophy—Symptoms & Causes*, n.d.).

TIPS FOR OVERCOMING AND RELIEVING VAGINAL ATROPHY

Managing vaginal atrophy involves lifestyle changes, medical treatments, and natural remedies. Below are some strategies:

- Give up smoking: Giving up smoking improves blood circulation and overall vaginal health.
- Stay sexually active: Regular sexual activity, including intercourse and masturbation, increases blood flow to the vaginal area and helps maintain tissue elasticity.
- Avoid scented feminine products: Use mild, unscented soaps. Avoid douches and feminine sprays that cause irritation.
- Exercise: Regular physical activity improves circulation, including to the vaginal tissues.
- Keep well hydrated: Staying hydrated helps maintain the health of mucous membranes, including those in the vagina.
- Natural lubricants: Using natural lubricants can alleviate dryness and discomfort during intercourse. Examples include:

    - Aloe vera gel: Soothes and moisturizes the vaginal area.
    - Coconut oil: A natural, hypoallergenic lubricant that provides long-lasting moisture.
    - Olive oil: Another natural option that can be used safely for lubrication.

In addition to these lifestyle changes, medical treatments like vaginal estrogen creams, tablets, or rings can be very effective. It's important to discuss all options with your doctor to find the most suitable treatment for you.

Understanding and addressing vaginal atrophy allows you to take control of your vaginal health and improve your overall well-being during and after menopause.

HAVING GREAT SEX DURING MENOPAUSE

The host of changes menopause makes to a woman's body can affect sexual health and satisfaction. But, with the right approach and some adjustments, it is possible to maintain and even enhance your sex life during this transition. Here are some strategies to help you have great sex during menopause:

WAYS TO INCREASE YOUR SEX DRIVE

Reduce Dryness With Moisturizers and Lubricants

One of the most common issues women face during this time is vaginal dryness, which can make sex uncomfortable or even painful. Using vaginal moisturizers and lubricants regularly can significantly reduce dryness, making intercourse more comfortable and fun. There are a variety of products available, including water-based and silicone-based lubricants, which can be tailored to your personal preferences and needs.

Talk to Your Partner About What You Like

Open communication with your partner is essential for a satisfying sex life. Discussing your likes, dislikes, and any concerns can help both of you feel more connected and comfortable. These conversations can also prompt you to try new things in the bedroom, which can reignite passion and excitement. Keep in mind that your partner may not be aware of the changes you're experiencing, so sharing as much information as you can may help them better understand and support you.

Get More Rest

Fatigue can be a barrier to a healthy sex life. Ensuring you get adequate rest can improve your overall energy levels and mood, making you more inclined to engage in sexual activity. Fostering a sleep routine, creating a restful sleeping environment, and addressing any sleep disturbances are steps you can take toward feeling more rested and ready for intimacy.

Schedule Time for Sex

Busy schedules and the demands of daily life can sometimes push sex to the bottom of your priority list. Scheduling time for sex can ensure that it remains an important part of your relationship. It doesn't have to be spontaneous to be fun; anticipating a romantic evening or a weekend getaway can build excitement and make the experience more special.

Spend More Time on Foreplay

Menopause can affect arousal and make it take longer for you to become fully aroused. Spending more time on foreplay can help increase arousal and ensure that you are both fully engaged and ready for intercourse. This can be kissing, touching, oral sex, or any other activities that you and your partner enjoy. The key is to take your time and focus on the pleasurable aspects of the experience.

Think About Sex

Did you know that your brain is a powerful sexual organ? Thinking about sex throughout the day can help increase your libido. You can achieve this by reading erotic literature, watching romantic or sexual content, or simply fantasizing about past intimate moments. Keeping your mind engaged with sexual thoughts can make you more receptive and excited about the prospect of sex.

Change Course From Intercourse

Sex doesn't always have to mean intercourse. Exploring other forms of sexual activity, like mutual masturbation, oral sex, or using sex toys, can provide you pleasure without the discomfort that may come with vaginal dryness or other symptoms. These activities can also add variety and excitement to your sex life, making it more fulfilling.

Reignite the Spark—Get Out of Your Sexual Rut

If your sex life has become monotonous, it might be time to shake things up. Try new positions, explore different locations, or incorporate fantasies or role-playing to help reignite the spark. Being open to experimenting can bring a sense of adventure and novelty to your sexual relationship, keeping it vibrant and satisfying.

Implementing these strategies puts you in a position to overcome some of the common challenges that menopause can present and continue to enjoy a fulfilling and exciting sex life. The key is to stay connected with your partner, communicate openly, and be willing to explore new ways to experience pleasure.

CAN YOU DATE DURING MENOPAUSE?

Navigating the dating world during this time can be both challenging and empowering. While the midlife dating game might feel intimidating because of the changes your body and emotions are undergoing, menopause can actually provide unique benefits that enhance your dating experience. Let's delve into why dating during menopause can be advantageous and offer practical tips to boost your confidence and enjoyment.

WHY THE MIDLIFE DATING GAME CAN FEEL INTIMIDATING

Dating at any age can be daunting, but midlife dating comes with its own set of challenges. The physical and emotional changes brought on by menopause can affect self-esteem and body image. Also, the social dynamics of dating might have shifted since the last time you were single, and this unfamiliar landscape can feel overwhelming. Concerns about sexual performance, societal perceptions of aging, and the fear of rejection can also contribute to the anxiety surrounding midlife dating.

WHY MENOPAUSE CAN ACTUALLY BE BENEFICIAL FOR DATING

Despite the challenges, menopause can bring a wealth of benefits to your dating life. Many women have a clearer sense of self and what they want in a partner at this stage of life. The wisdom and experience gained over the years can lead to more authentic and fulfilling relationships. Also, the end of reproductive concerns can free you from the anxieties of contraception and the potential for pregnancy, allowing for a more relaxed and spontaneous approach to sex and intimacy.

TIPS FOR DATING DURING MENOPAUSE

- Wear an outfit you trust: You can boost your confidence by wearing an outfit that makes you feel comfortable and attractive. Choose clothing that fits well, highlights your best features, and aligns with your personal style. Feeling good about how you look can set a positive tone for the date and help you focus on enjoying the experience rather than worrying about your looks.
- Meet a friend beforehand: Meeting a friend before your date can help get rid of pre-date jitters. A chat with someone you trust can boost your morale and provide a reassuring start to the evening. They can also boost your confidence, reminding you of your strengths and why you deserve a great partner.
- Avoid alcohol: It might be tempting to have a drink to calm your nerves, but alcohol can sometimes exacerbate symptoms like hot flashes and mood swings. It can also impair judgment and hinder a genuine connection. Opt for non-alcoholic beverages that keep you hydrated and clear-headed.
- Plan active dates: Doing activities can take the pressure off the constant conversation and create opportunities for genuine interactions. It could be a walk in the park, a museum visit, or

a cooking class. Active dates can be fun and much less stressful. They also give you a shared experience to bond over and can highlight common interests.

- Boost your sexual confidence: Menopause can affect your sexual confidence, but it's important to remember that sexual satisfaction often improves with open communication and understanding. Educate yourself about your changing body and explore new ways to enjoy intimacy. Lubricants and vaginal moisturizers can enhance comfort, and talking to a healthcare professional can offer additional solutions.
- Remember you aren't the only one: It's easy to feel isolated in your experiences, but many others are navigating the same challenges. Remembering that you're not alone is reassuring. Support groups, both online and offline, can provide a sense of community and shared understanding.
- Communication is key: Open and honest communication with potential partners is crucial. Sharing your experiences with menopause can foster intimacy and understanding. It can also help set realistic expectations and reduce misunderstandings. Being upfront about your needs and boundaries can lead to more respectful and fulfilling relationships.

Menopause does not signify the end of dating or sexual enjoyment. On the contrary, it can be a time of rediscovery and new beginnings. If you are single, you should feel encouraged to go out, have fun, and seek meaningful connections if that is what you want. Embracing this phase of life with confidence and an open heart can lead to fulfilling and enriching dating experiences. Remember, dating during this time is not about conforming to societal expectations but about finding joy, companionship, and love on your own terms.

DELVING INTO INTIMACY

The changes that menopause brings about make significant changes to a woman's body, and these can impact sexual experiences. But this doesn't signify the end of a fulfilling, intimate life. Let's delve into the journey of a woman who navigated the challenges of menopause and emerged with a deeper, more satisfying connection with her partner. Her story illustrates how perseverance, communication, and adaptation can sustain and even enhance intimacy during and after menopause.

Lauren's Journey Through Menopausal Intimacy

Lauren had always enjoyed a robust and satisfying sex life with her partner, Mark. But, as she entered her late 40s and the early stages of menopause, she started experiencing some sexual problems that affected their intimacy. "It was like my body had betrayed me," she recalled. "The dryness, the discomfort, and the lack of desire—it was all so frustrating." These changes took a toll on her confidence and left her feeling disconnected from Mark.

Determined not to let menopause drive a wedge between them, Lauren and Mark decided to face these challenges head-on. They began by educating themselves about the physical changes she was experiencing. Understanding that decreased estrogen levels were behind her symptoms, they explored various solutions to mitigate the effects.

One of the first strategies they employed was using lubricants and vaginal moisturizers. "It was a simple fix, but it made a world of difference," she noted. These products alleviated dryness and discomfort, making sexual activities more enjoyable. They also experimented with different brands and types until they found the ones that worked best for them.

Communication was another big element in their approach. Lauren and Mark had candid conversations about their needs and concerns. "Talking about it openly was key," she emphasized. "It wasn't always easy, but it brought us closer." These discussions helped them to remain empathetic and patient with each other.

Lauren also focused on her overall well-being. She made sure she got enough rest, stayed active, and practiced stress-reducing activities like yoga and meditation. These lifestyle changes had a positive impact on her libido and energy levels.

Another strategy was redefining intimacy beyond intercourse. Lauren and Mark spent more time on foreplay and exploring other forms of physical affection. "We discovered new ways to connect," she said. "It wasn't just about the end goal but about enjoying each other in different ways." This shift in focus helped them maintain a fulfilling intimate relationship even when traditional intercourse was less frequent.

The turning point came when Lauren and Mark took a weekend getaway to reconnect. "We decided to leave behind the pressures of daily life and just focus on each other," she shared. The break allowed them to relax and reignite their passion. "It was like we found each other all over again," she smiled. This experience marked the moment when they truly felt their sex life had bounced back.

Lauren's optimism about her sex life during menopause was rooted in her belief that intimacy is a journey rather than a destination. She advises other women to maintain a positive outlook and to be proactive in addressing any challenges. "Menopause doesn't have to mean the end of your sex life," she affirmed. "With the right mindset and support, it can be a time of rediscovery and deeper connection."

HOW TO BE OPTIMISTIC ABOUT SEX LIFE DURING MENOPAUSE

1. Educate yourself: Understanding the changes your body is going through can demystify and destigmatize them. Knowledge is empowering and can guide you towards solutions that work for you.
2. Communicate openly: Conversing with your partner about your experiences and needs fosters intimacy and reduces misunderstandings. A supportive partner makes a big difference.
3. Experiment with different solutions: Don't be afraid to try different products or methods to find what works best for you. Lubricants, moisturizers, and other aids can increase comfort and pleasure.
4. Focus on overall health: Maintaining good physical and mental health can improve your libido and energy levels. Regular exercise, sufficient sleep, and stress management are needed.
5. Redefine intimacy: Intimacy is not solely about intercourse. Exploring other forms of affection and connection can sustain and enrich your relationship.
6. Stay positive and patient: Changes don't happen overnight. Keeping a positive attitude and being patient with yourself and your partner can make the journey smoother and more rewarding.

Lauren's story is a testament to the resilience and adaptability one needs to maintain intimacy during menopause. By embracing change and finding new ways to connect, you can continue to enjoy a fulfilling and vibrant sex life well into your menopausal years.

Navigating the changes in your sex life during menopause can be challenging, but it is entirely manageable with the right knowledge and strategies. Understanding that vaginal dryness, bladder changes, low sexual desire, and body image concerns are common can help normalize these experiences and encourage proactive management. Making use of lubricants, practicing pelvic floor exercises, maintaining open communication with your partner, and seeking professional help when needed are practical steps to enhance intimacy. Also, recognizing the symptoms and treatment options for vaginal atrophy is crucial for maintaining vaginal health. Embracing these changes and exploring new ways to connect with your partner can lead to a fulfilling, intimate life. As we move forward, it's important to remember that menopause affects various aspects of your well-being, including your hair. In the next chapter, we will explore how hormonal changes impact your hair and provide tips for keeping your locks healthy and vibrant, continuing our journey to empower you through this transformative phase.

LET'S TALK HAIR

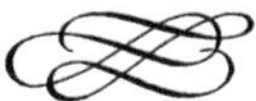

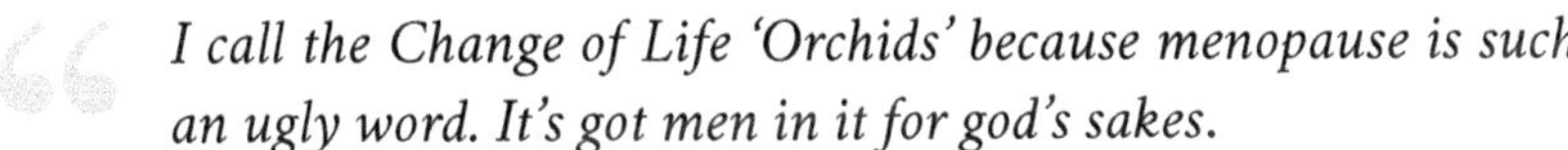

I call the Change of Life 'Orchids' because menopause is such an ugly word. It's got men in it for god's sakes.

— LISA JEY DAVIS

As we transition through menopause, we may encounter a range of physical changes, one of the most noticeable being alterations in hair health. Menopause, marked by a decline in estrogen levels, can lead to hair thinning, breakage, and changes in texture. Understanding how menopause affects hair can empower us to take proactive steps in maintaining hair vitality and embracing this stage of life with confidence and grace.

HOW DOES MENOPAUSE AFFECT YOUR HAIR?

Many women notice that their hair gets thinner and shorter throughout menopause. Estrogen promotes hair growth, and menopause lowers estrogen levels, which is why this happens.

Your hair may break more easily during menopause. This is a result of your scalp producing weaker, thinner new hair.

Menopause can result in even more hair thinning for women whose hair is sensitive to the hormone DHT. Less estrogen means more testosterone, which can damage hair follicles and cause hair thinning.

Symptoms of Menopausal Hair Thinning

Hair thinning is gradual. So, even though the average age for the onset of menopause is 50, changes in hair can start before then. Below are some changes you may notice:

- You have a thinner ponytail.
- Your parting is wider, and your hair is not growing as long as it once did.
- You may see more of your scalp around your head's crown.
- Receding in your temple area
- Density decreases at the frontal hairline
- A decrease in each strand's length and thickness.

Hair loss can make you feel self-conscious, but the saving grace is it is not permanent. Here are some tips on how to mitigate hair thinning.

Tips for Reducing Hair Thinning

Reduce Stress

Managing your stress levels can help you prevent hormonal imbalance. The decrease in estrogen production alters brain chemistry and can lead to mood swings, anxiety, and apathy. Practicing yoga and other forms of breathing relaxation are particularly effective in combating the symptoms of menopause. Regular exercise is another good way to lower stress.

Be Active

Once you incorporate exercise into your routine, you'll feel stronger and happier. You can use it to prevent several other symptoms like weight gain, mood swings, and insomnia.

Choose an exercise regimen that suits your needs. You could try running, joining a gym, or going for walks with a friend.

Eat Well

Consuming a well-balanced, low-fat diet is the most effective way to prevent hair loss. You can achieve it by making sure that all your meals have sufficient fruits, vegetables, and whole grains. You should also include mono-saturated oils like olive and sesame oil.

Should you want to supplement your diet, you can try drinking green tea, taking folic acid and vitamin B6 supplements, and consuming foods that contain essential fatty acids.

The following foods contain fatty acids:

- almonds
- flaxseed oil
- salmon
- tuna
- walnuts

Stay Hydrated

Drink plenty of water throughout the day and cut back on juices, sodas, and other flavored drinks that have more sugar than is necessary for your body. Individual needs for water consumption differ and are influenced by a number of variables, like level of physical activity and general health. Generally speaking, though, you should aim for eight eight-ounce glasses of water every day.

Keep It Natural

Avoid using heat, like hair dryers and straighteners, to avoid drying out and breaking your hair. Extensions and other styling techniques can also weaken the hair and speed up hair loss.

If you must dye your hair, opt for natural dye because the artificial chemicals used in perms and dyes might harm the hair and scalp.

Always use a nourishing conditioner after washing your hair to maintain the health of your scalp and encourage healthy hair development.

Wearing a swimming cap is recommended if you swim, as chlorine can cause hair breakage, and a sun hat will prevent your hair from drying out and breaking when you spend a lot of time outside in the sun or wind.

#1 SECRET TO THICK, HEALTHY HAIR: USING AN OIL MASSAGE

Retaining thick, healthy hair can be as simple as incorporating a regular oil massage into your hair care routine. It's an age-old secret that has been cherished for its ability to nourish the scalp, promote blood circulation, and strengthen hair follicles, resulting in luscious, vibrant hair.

Hair oiling is applying oil to hair and rubbing it into the scalp to boost hydration, sheen, and shine. Regular hair washing strips the hair of its vitamins and minerals, so oiling can help restore these.

How to Oil Your Hair

1. Use your fingertips to massage oil into your scalp in a circular motion.
2. Distribute the oil left on your palms onto the rest of your hair.
3. Put a shower cap or towel over it and leave it on overnight.
4. Shampoo hair when it's dry, then give it a good rinse.

5. Condition as usual, or use coconut oil as a conditioner.

Which Oils to Use

Your hair's needs will determine which oil you use; as different oils contain different vitamins.

- atlas cedarwood oil
- bay Leaf
- chamomile
- clary sage
- lemon oil
- peppermint oil
- rosemary oil
- thyme oil
- ylang ylang oil

HOW TO OIL YOUR HAIR SAFELY

- Always do a patch test.
- Be mindful of the concentration of essential oils.
- Be aware of any allergies you have.

DIY MOISTURE HAIR MASKS

Do-it-yourself treatments are a wise decision for several reasons:

- Cost-effectiveness: Specialized therapies can be costly, so treating your hair at home can save you a lot of money in the long term.
- You have control over what goes on in your hair: You can be certain of what you're putting on your hair and scalp when you DIY. If you are allergic to anything or have sensitivities, you can easily avoid it.

- Flexibility: The best thing about doing it yourself is that you can modify the recipes to suit your own needs.

Here is a list of carefully selected homemade remedies that you can quickly make and apply. They are made to specifically address the hair care issues that menopausal women face.

Silken Essence Hair Elixir

Ingredients:

- 2 tablespoons of coconut oil
- 1 tablespoon of Proactive rosemary hair booster oil

Instructions:

1. To make the oil mixture, first combine the oils in a small bowl. To improve the absorption into your hair and scalp, warm it up a little.
2. Apply to Hair and Scalp: If your hair is long or thick, part it and then evenly distribute the oils from roots to ends. The rosemary oil improves hair health and stimulates the scalp, and the coconut oil offers intense nourishment.
3. Apply and Massage: For a few minutes, use your fingertips to gently massage the oils into your scalp. This enhances blood circulation and can lead to better hair growth and general scalp health. Make sure the oil is spread evenly throughout the strands of your hair.
4. Give the oil mixture time to penetrate by letting it sit on your scalp for at least half an hour. This lets the oils' nutritious qualities fully permeate your hair and condition it from the inside out.
5. Shampoo and Rinse: To get rid of the oil residue, give your hair a thorough wash with a mild shampoo. To make sure all

of the oil is properly rinsed out, you might need to shampoo twice.

6. Optional: Condition: Use a conditioner after shampooing if you want more smoothness or if your hair tends to be dry. Apply the conditioner only to your hair's mid-lengths to ends, avoiding the area of your scalp where the oils were applied.
7. Style as Desired: After washing and conditioning your hair, style it as you normally would. After this nourishing treatment, your hair will probably feel softer, appear shinier, and be easier to manage.

Golden Nourish-Avo Hair Mask

Ingredients:

- 1 tablespoon of Proactive Rosemary hair oil
- 1 medium avocado
- 2 tablespoons of raw honey

Instructions:

1. Get the mask ready: Slice the avocado in half, extract the pit, and transfer the meat to a mixing dish. Blend the avocado until it's creamy and lump-free.
2. Add the oil and honey: Stir the honey into the avocado. Honey is ideal for moisturizing dry or damaged hair since it is a natural humectant, which means it draws and holds moisture. Add the Proactive rosemary hair booster oil next. This combination not only moisturizes hair but also feeds the scalp and encourages healthy growth.
3. Mix: Blend the oil, honey, and mashed avocado until you get a smooth and creamy texture. Blend thoroughly to maximize the benefits.

4. Apply: Part your hair and evenly apply the mask from the roots to the ends. Concentrate on rubbing it onto your scalp as well.
5. Rest: After applying the mask, let it sit in your hair for 40 to 50 minutes. This way, it can penetrate your hair shaft and offer hydration and repair.
6. Shampoo and Rinse: Give your hair a thorough rinse with warm water. Continue with your typical wash and conditioner regimen after that.

MANAGING UNWANTED FACIAL HAIR

The positives that come with menopause are fewer legs and underarm hair. But on the flip side, it's also the stage where coarse, dark hairs on the jawline, chin, or upper lip may begin to appear. For some women, it feels like the last blow to their femininity and makes them feel shame.

What Causes It?

The fall in estrogen levels and fluctuations in testosterone levels cause hair growth.

How to Manage It

There's nothing you can do to stop the onset, but there are ways to reduce it so you can feel better about the way you look.

1. Apply cream: Depilatory creams have advanced significantly. However, some women are sensitive to the chemicals that break down hair, so always do a quick patch test on a different area of your body to see if there are any reactions.
2. Shave: Shaving is an inexpensive and practical solution. To avoid rashes or ingrown hair, shave during or shortly after a shower when the hair is softer. Use a sharp razor.

3. Pull them out: If there are just a few, you can pull them out with tweezers. Contrary to popular belief, tweezing will not make your hair grow back coarser or darker. If you have a bit more hair, you can try threading or waxing. To avoid ingrown hair, both procedures should be carried out by professionals.
4. Laser hair removal: The laser beams damage the follicle by overheating it, which prevents hair growth. The results are long-lasting, but it can be a tad costly depending on the extent of the work needed and where you live. It may also take numerous sessions. Laser hair removal is ineffective on fine or light-colored hair.
5. Electrolysis: Electrolysis targets one hair at a time. A tiny probe is inserted straight into the hair follicle, where it is heated to the point of devastation by a low-level electrical current. It can cause minor pain and possibly scarring. It may take up to 18 months to achieve the desired outcomes, but it is permanent and suitable for any color of hair.

CARING FOR YOUR SKIN DURING MENOPAUSE

How Menopause Can Affect the Skin

- sun damage and age spots
- dry skin
- easy bruising
- acne or pimple
- rashes and sensitive skin
- jowls, wrinkles, and slack skin
- slow healing

Skin Care Tips

- Use a gentle cleanser containing ceramides, hyaluronic acid, glycerin, and warm water to wash your face.

- Apply a moisturizer containing glycerin, hyaluronic acid, or ceramides.
- Put SPF 30 sunblock on.
- Before going to bed, use the same cleanser and a peptide-rich anti-aging product.

In the journey through menopause, changes in hair quality can be a challenging aspect for many women. The decline in estrogen levels triggers a cascade of effects on hair thickness, length, and resilience. However, understanding these changes and adopting proactive measures can greatly alleviate concerns. From managing stress and staying active to embracing natural hair care practices and exploring DIY hair treatments, there's a wealth of strategies to support hair health during this transition. By nurturing both body and mind, you can navigate menopausal hair changes with confidence, knowing that, with care and patience, healthy hair is within reach.

Speaking of nurturing the body and mind, let's tackle another very important aspect regarding health: getting a good night's rest.

EMBRACING MENOPAUSE – WITHOUT THE MYSTERY!

"Menopause is not the end; it's a new beginning. Embrace the changes, and you'll find the strength within."

— ANONYMOUS

Menopause is a completely natural part of life that every woman must go through, yet many women find it difficult and destabilizing. When you're losing sleep and your memory's foggy, and your body doesn't feel like something you recognize anymore, it can easily feel like you're losing yourself. But it doesn't have to be this way, and when you're properly prepared and know how to navigate every symptom as it arises, it's a very different story.

This is knowledge that every woman should have access to, yet discussion about menopause has been silenced for such a long time, that remarkably few of us really know what to expect or how to handle it. This book is designed to bridge that gap in understanding, empowering more women to step into this new phase of life with confidence – and without ever losing sight of who they are.

Now that you're halfway through, you're invited to join the mission to help more women navigate menopause with positivity and confidence – and the great news is, that all it takes is for you to leave a short review.

By leaving a review of this book on Amazon, you'll show new readers where they can find this life-changing guidance for addressing the symptoms of menopause naturally.

There are so many women looking for information about how to navigate menopause, and your review will help them find it quickly and easily.

Thank you so much for your support. It's amazing what we can do when we work together.

Scan the QR code below

SLEEPING SOUNDLY

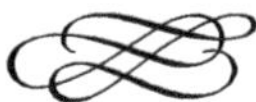

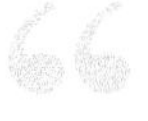

I believe whole-heartedly that age is a mindset. Biological age is what it is, but I truly believe it's more about how you feel - how you feel in your body and how you feel about your body.

— JENNIFER GREY

POOR SLEEP AND MENOPAUSE

Menopause symptoms can endure for years beyond one's final menstrual cycle, and they often start four to seven years beforehand. Multiple sleep disorders can be caused by hormonal changes, bodily changes, and life changes that occur during this time.

Insomnia

People are more likely to develop insomnia during and after the menopausal transition. Insomnia actually makes you more aware of the hot flashes and night sweats you would otherwise sleep through.

Insomnia during menopause can also be caused by anxiety and depression. Hormonal imbalance and the life changes that come with getting older can lead to deteriorating mental health. Most people who experience anxiety or depression report chronic sleeplessness (Pacheco, 2021).

Hot Flashes and Night Sweats

Hot flashes, or night sweats, are periods of extreme warmth that radiate upward from the chest. They typically last two to four minutes and are usually accompanied by anxiety and heavy perspiration. The pain and agitation that wakes one up during a hot flash can make it more difficult for them to get back to sleep. As we approach menopause, we tend to have more regular night sweats, which might continue to happen frequently and intensely in the years right after our final period.

Sleep Apnea and Snoring

Reproductive hormone decline can cause soft tissues in the neck to become more easily collapsed, and menopausal weight gain can exacerbate blockages in the airways. This results in snoring and a disruption in sleep patterns.

Snoring may indicate the presence of sleep apnea, a condition that causes brief intervals of shallow or nonexistent breathing. These breathing episodes have the potential to worsen long-term physical and mental health issues, impair sleep quality, and cause drowsiness during the day. Sleep apnea affects around a quarter of adults in the years leading up to menopause and more than a third in the years that follow (Pacheco, 2021).

Restless Legs Syndrome

Restless legs syndrome, or RLS, is a sleep disorder that produces painful sensations in the legs when lying down. It affects more than half of post-menopausal women. Experts speculate that after menopause, iron deficiency and changing hormones may cause RLS. Movement usually relieves this discomfort, but only momentarily, which might interfere with sleep and perhaps result in insomnia (Derwent, 2022).

WHY DOES MENOPAUSE AFFECT SLEEP?

The body produces less progesterone and estrogen throughout the menopausal transition. Those happen to be the two hormones essential to the reproductive cycle. Various bodily systems and functions are then impacted by these changes, including a number that has an effect on sleep, namely:

- Metabolism: Menopause impacts the way food is broken down into energy. Low estrogen levels have been linked to weight gain, which is linked to the emergence of sleep apnea or snoring.
- Circadian Rhythm: Many women experience a deterioration of their circadian rhythms after menopause.
- Thermoregulation: As estrogen levels drop, the brain becomes more sensitive to changes in body temperature. In an attempt to cool itself, the body initiates processes like sweating at lower temperatures, and this results in hot flashes and night sweats.
- Mood: The neurotransmitters involved in mood regulation can be disrupted by changes in estrogen levels. This is why mood swings, anxiety, and depression are more common during the menopausal transition, as well as the sleep issues that go along with them.

Creating an optimal sleep environment is crucial for quality rest and overall well-being.

HOW TO OPTIMIZE YOUR SLEEP ENVIRONMENT

Temperature

While some people sleep relatively coolly, others run hot in bed. Nonetheless, during sleep, the body temperature of every healthy adult drops. This is because a lower core temperature makes you feel drowsy, and a higher temperature keeps you awake.

Experts agree that 65° F, or 18° C, is the perfect bedroom temperature for sleeping, regardless of whether you sleep under a thick quilt or just a top sheet. A colder thermostat setting helps you keep your core temperature low as you sleep.

However, not everyone finds 65 degrees to be the ideal temperature. Try adding a layer or two to your bedding if you think it is too chilly. If you feel warmer, think about taking a layer off or switching to lighter bed linens.

Noise

A quieter bedroom is preferable for optimal sleep. Your physical and mental health could suffer from extreme sleep disruption and fragmentation brought on by loud noise disturbances. Low-level noise may even lead you to transition into a lighter sleep stage or to wake up briefly.

You can keep your room quiet by blocking outside noise to the best of your ability. You can use a fan or a white noise machine. Some people even listen to ambient sounds or relaxing music before bed. It is said to reduce feelings of anxiety and ease physical discomfort.

Light

Your circadian rhythms, which govern your sleep-wake cycle, are greatly impacted by natural light and darkness. Your eyes detect sunlight during the day, which prompts the brain to release the hormone cortisol, which keeps you awake and energized. Your brain then releases the hormone melatonin when darkness descends at night, which promotes feelings of relaxation and drowsiness.

When you are exposed to artificial light in the evening, it might cause a delay in your circadian rhythms and increase the amount of time it takes you to fall asleep.

Lux units are used to measure light intensity. Research indicates that exposure to light sources with a lux level of 10 or higher later in the day can cause a decrease in slow-wave sleep, which is an essential part of your sleep cycle for body restoration and cell repair. They can also cause you to wake up in the night. Even with nighttime screen settings, the artificial blue light from smartphones, televisions, and other screens can be harmful to your sleep (Perry, 2021).

If you enjoy reading in bed before going to sleep, try keeping the lights in your room as low as possible. Dimmable lighting will facilitate a more restful night's sleep. Minimize screens in your bedroom, especially televisions.

Mattress and Bedding

You might like the soft support of latex, the near-body shape of memory foam, or the bouncy feel of a coil mattress, depending on your sleeping preferences. Research suggests that modern mattresses reduce back discomfort and improve sleep quality. The ideal mattress for you, however, probably varies depending on personal characteristics like body weight, preferred firmness or softness of surface, and typical sleeping posture (Pacheco, 2021).

It's best to choose your bedding according to personal preferences. Take into account the cushion, firmness, thickness, and durability of the mattress. The ideal choice for sheets could depend on how hot you sleep at night and if you like a crisp or silky feeling.

Lastly, maintaining a clean bedroom is essential for encouraging sound sleep. Dust mites cause allergies, so you can reduce their prevalence by vacuuming your carpet and cleaning your bedding on a regular basis. To prevent damage or excessive shrinkage, just make sure you follow the washing and drying recommendations on the care tags of your bedding.

TIPS FOR BETTER SLEEP HYGIENE

Even though menopause is unavoidable, women can still take steps to enhance the quality of their sleep:

Take a Cool Shower Before Bed

A shower a couple of hours before bed cools you down and promotes sound sleep. It feels good to wash off the day, even if you showered that morning.

You're usually pressed for time in the morning, so taking a shower at night gives you the luxury of leisure. If you have a lot of trouble with insomnia, consider helping unwind your body and mind before taking a bath or shower by taking a sleeping pill.

Wear Lightweight, Breathable Cotton Clothes

Menopausal women are advised to dress in lightweight, breathable cotton clothing since it helps to control body temperature and enhance comfort. Cotton has better ventilation, which may lessen the severity of hot flashes and night sweats. Cotton is also soft on the skin, minimizing irritation and enhancing general skin health. During this time of life, wearing loose-fitting cotton clothing can also give you a sense of freedom and flexibility of movement, which will make your everyday activities more pleasant.

Sleep With Light Covers

Menopausal women benefit from sleeping with light covers because of the frequent changes in body temperature. Light covers, like light blankets or sheets, improve airflow and heat dissipation, lessening discomfort and overheating at night. Since thick blankets or duvets can exacerbate hot flashes and night sweats, this can be especially useful for women experiencing these symptoms. Choosing lighter coverings results in a more pleasant sleeping environment, which, in turn, leads to more restful evenings and fewer disturbances from temperature changes.

Use a Fan or Air Conditioning

Menopausal women can effectively regulate the fluctuations in body temperature and encourage better sleep by using fans or air conditioning. Circulated air has a cooling effect that helps reduce night sweats and hot flashes. In a similar vein, air conditioning lowers the risk of overheating at night by maintaining a reasonable room temperature. This creates a more comfortable resting environment that promotes unbroken and restful nights.

Be Consistent With Bedtime

Establishing a healthy sleep schedule is crucial, and that requires consistency with bedtime. The body's internal clock becomes regulated when a routine is followed. This means sleeping and waking up at reasonable times. A regular bedtime can help with trouble sleeping by encouraging deeper, more restorative sleep cycles. Calming activities will help with healthy and consistent sleep.

CREATE A RELAXING BEDTIME ROUTINE EACH NIGHT

Set an Alarm

Using an Android smartphone app or an iPhone sleep timer, you can set an alarm or notification on your phone. It will serve as a helpful cue to switch off and get ready for bed.

Eat Light and Healthy Before Bed

Alcohol consumption and late dining might promote weight gain and create bad sleeping patterns. To increase your metabolism and get better sleep, try cutting your eating window down to 10 hours a day. If you do experience late-night cravings, consider eating healthier foods like almonds, yogurt, or oatmeal to increase your melatonin levels before going to bed. Having a dessert or nightcap in the evening can be detrimental to your sleep. Due to its depressive properties, alcohol can induce sleepiness, but the effects wear off fast, throwing off your circadian rhythm and reducing melatonin levels, which delays REM sleep. If you consume alcohol late on a regular basis, your tolerance grows, and more alcohol is needed to achieve drowsiness.

Curate a Pre-Bedtime Playlist

Creating a playlist to be played before bed can help you decompress and release the mental attachments of the day. Listening to music, especially classical music, might improve sleep. However, you are not obligated to listen to a specific genre. Listen to whatever you like as long as it's somewhat calming.

Aside from music, there are also effective new developments in audio sleep aids. Color noises are artificially produced sound waves with brain-interacting frequencies. White noise, for instance, sounds like snow on a TV screen. Pink noise is gentler. Brown noise has an ocean-like depth and calming quality.

Try Quick Foam Rolling or a Yoga Session

Before going to bed, try foam rolling and yoga to help unwind your muscles and center your thoughts. They release tension, slow down the body and mind, and enhance the quality of sleep.

Foam rolling, sometimes referred to as trigger point therapy or myofascial release, helps alleviate stiffness and tightness in the muscles. It improves blood flow as well, much like a massage.

Yoga is good for centering yourself. The various poses release tension from the lower back, shoulders, and hamstrings. They also release tension from muscles you never even realized were tight. Play your bedtime playlist as you engage for optimal effects.

Drink Something Warm

A warm beverage before bed can make you feel comfortable and ready for bed. For millennia, people have used chamomile tea to curb insomnia and sleep problems.

Turmeric is a superfood that promotes restful sleep, reduces inflammation and depression, and eases pain. It is available at your neighborhood farmer's market or grocery shop. It is a tad bitter, so consider making a soothing drink like turmeric golden milk to lessen its bitterness.

Use Aromatherapy Oils

Aromatherapy and essential oils are used to help manage stress. You can use these oils in a diffuser or apply them directly on your skin.

They are often used by intensive care patients as an alternative to sleep-inducing drugs. Before tucking yourself in, try adding a little lavender and cedar oil to your diffuser.

Aromatherapy and essential oils might not be for everyone, particularly those with allergies or odor sensitivity, but it's still worth a try.

Your bedtime routine shouldn't be too lengthy. 30–60 minutes is good. It gives you plenty of time to relax without feeling pressed for time. The aim is to build consistency. It will prepare your body for sleep and promote productivity the following day.

A nightly routine can assist you in winding down and ending the day. After unwinding and getting ready for bed, settle into your cozy mattress, grab your go-to pillow, and drift off to sleep.

LIFESTYLE CHANGES FOR BETTER SLEEP

Limit Your Caffeine Intake

Caffeine's effects linger for three to seven hours. So consuming it before bedtime could lead to staying awake for longer than you'd like. It's advisable to restrict your caffeine intake to the morning but keep in mind that tolerance varies from person to person. Some can stop in the afternoon; others need to stop a lot earlier in order to get sleep. The less you consume, the more susceptible you are to its effects.

Go to Bed Only When You Are Tired

Try not to lie in bed tossing and turning if you aren't tired. Opt for a soothing pastime until you are tired, and then you can get into bed. If you lie awake for 20 minutes or longer, get out. Because the feeling of being unable to fall asleep might lead to frustration or stress, both of which can prolong your awake time.

After getting out of bed, engage in a relaxing activity such as stretching or reading until you feel tired enough to go back to bed.

Manage Stress Before Going to Bed

Overthinking can keep you awake. To lessen the likelihood that your worries keep you awake:

- Write down your concerns to help release them from your mind.
- If your to-do list makes you anxious, do it at night. Set your priorities for the upcoming day and the remainder of the week, then make the effort to unwind.
- A weighted blanket can be as beneficial as deep-pressure therapy for treating anxiety and sleeplessness.
- Try meditation.

TIPS FOR RELIEF FROM NIGHT SWEATS

1. Flip your pillow.
2. Use a cooling gel pillow or put an ice pack under your pillow.
3. Keep an insulated water bottle filled with cold water near the bed.
4. Keep cooling spray by the bed.

Jennifer Grey's perspective resonates deeply with the challenges and triumphs of menopausal women, particularly concerning our sleep patterns. Age, as she suggests, is indeed a mindset, and how one feels in their body and about their body can significantly impact their quality of life during menopause. The journey through menopause can be tumultuous, marked by hormonal shifts that disrupt sleep and lead to various sleep disorders like insomnia, hot flashes, night sweats, and even restless legs syndrome. Understanding the physiological changes during menopause, such as hormonal imbalances affecting metabolism, circadian rhythms, thermoregulation, and mood regulation, sheds light on why sleep disturbances are prevalent during this stage of life. Implementing strategies to optimize the sleep environment, from managing temperature and noise to creating a relaxing bedtime routine and making lifestyle adjustments, can greatly improve sleep quality and overall well-being for menopausal women. By embracing a holistic approach that addresses physical, mental, and environmental factors, women can navigate menopause with resilience and a renewed focus on health and vitality. Now that sleep has been tackled, let's get into another big issue during menopause: memory loss and brain fog.

WHAT WAS I DOING AGAIN?

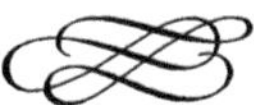

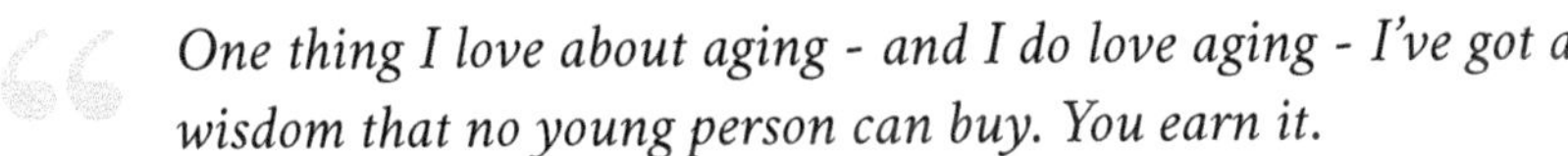

> *One thing I love about aging - and I do love aging - I've got a wisdom that no young person can buy. You earn it.*
>
> — SUZANNE SOMERS

THE TRUTH ABOUT MEMORY LOSS

Do you ever lose track of names, appointments, or your keys? You're not alone, so don't worry. Memory loss is part and parcel of perimenopause and menopause.

Even the sharpest people can become anxious and concerned that their brain's capacity is deteriorating due to forgetfulness. A lot of women are worried that this might be an early indication of dementia. Fortunately for most of us, it isn't.

Menopausal memory loss is typically mild. It might be hard to distinguish between memory loss associated with aging and menopause because memory declines gradually with age.

What Causes It?

Estrogen promotes the creation of new cells and facilitates the formation of new connections between existing cells by stimulating the brain and maintaining neural activity. Your entire body, including your brain, experiences an abrupt deprivation state when your estrogen levels drop.

The drop in estrogen levels can lead to forgetfulness. When it comes to mental processes like focus and memory, estrogen is essential. Women may suffer from cognitive symptoms like mental fog, inability to concentrate, and forgetfulness as their estrogen levels drop. This hormonal change may also have an impact on the brain's neurotransmitters, which may impair cell-to-cell communication and cause memory loss. Because menopause is also accompanied by mood swings, stress, and sleep disorders, it can also aggravate cognitive issues and forgetfulness.

THE DIFFERENCE BETWEEN BRAIN FOG AND MORE SERIOUS COGNITIVE DECLINE

Brain fog means mental haziness, difficulty concentrating, and forgetfulness. It can feel frustrating, but it's important to distinguish it from more serious cognitive decline.

Serious cognitive decline, like dementia or Alzheimer's disease, involves progressive and irreversible changes in brain structure and function. These conditions are characterized by persistent and worsening memory loss, confusion, disorientation, and difficulty performing daily tasks.

To differentiate between the two, consider these key factors:

1. Duration and Persistence: Brain fog is often intermittent and temporary, fluctuating with hormonal changes and lifestyle

factors, whereas cognitive decline is persistent and worsens over time.

2. Severity of Symptoms: Brain fog can cause mild forgetfulness and occasional lapses in concentration, whereas cognitive decline leads to significant memory impairment, affecting daily functioning and independence.
3. Underlying Causes: Brain fog is usually linked to hormonal shifts and menopausal symptoms, while cognitive decline stems from neurological conditions, genetics, or other medical factors.
4. Response to Interventions: Brain fog can often be managed and improved with lifestyle changes, like adequate sleep, stress reduction, a healthy diet, and brain exercises, whereas cognitive decline requires comprehensive medical evaluation and treatment.

Understanding the difference between the two empowers us to address cognitive changes effectively. Adopting a holistic approach that includes healthy habits, mental stimulation, and regular monitoring of cognitive function helps us navigate this transition with confidence and clarity of mind.

VITAMIN B12 DEFICIENCY AND BRAIN FOG

Vitamin B12, also known as cobalamin, plays a role in brain function and overall neurological health. When women are deficient in this essential vitamin, they experience a myriad of symptoms, one being brain fog. This is how the relationship between Vitamin B12 deficiency and brain fog works:

- Neurological Impact: Vitamin B12 is essential for the production of myelin, a protective sheath that surrounds nerve fibers. Myelin helps transmit nerve signals related to concentration, memory, and cognition. Vitamin B12 deficiency can disrupt myelin production, which leads to brain fog.

- Homocysteine Levels: Vitamin B12 helps with metabolizing the amino acid homocysteine. Vitamin B deficiency leads to elevated levels of homocysteine, and that can impair blood flow to the brain, leading to brain fog.
- Neurotransmitter Function: Vitamin B12 is also involved in the synthesis of neurotransmitters like serotonin and dopamine, which play key roles in mood regulation and cognitive function. A Vitamin B12 deficiency can disrupt the balance of neurotransmitters, leading to symptoms like brain fog, mood swings, and memory impairment.
- Anemia and Oxygen Delivery: A deficiency in vitamin B12 can lead to megaloblastic anemia. It is an enlargement of immature red blood cells. It reduces the oxygen-carrying capacity of the blood, affecting brain function and contributing to fatigue, confusion, and brain fog.

Understanding the symptoms of a vitamin B12 shortage is essential for prompt intervention.

Signs of Vitamin B12 Deficiency

- Fatigue: This is due to the reduced oxygen-carrying capacity of the blood.
- Pale Skin: This is caused by megaloblastic anemia.
- Poor Mood: This includes feelings of irritability, depression, and anxiety.
- Sore and Red Tongue: This is called glossitis; it is a common oral symptom of B12 deficiency.
- Pins and Needles: Numbness or tingling sensations in the hands or feet.
- Memory and Concentration Problems: Brain fog, forgetfulness, and difficulty focusing.

Vitamin B12 deficiency is particularly common in women experiencing menopause. Hormonal changes can affect nutrient absorption in the digestive tract, leading to deficiencies in essential vitamins and minerals. Also, women in this phase of life may have dietary restrictions or changes that impact their B12 intake, like a reduced consumption of animal products or changes in nutrient absorption due to age-related factors.

Diagnosis and Treatment

Diagnosis typically involves blood tests to measure Vitamin B12 levels and assess markers like homocysteine and methylmalonic acid. Treatment often includes Vitamin B12 supplements, either orally or via injections, to replenish deficient levels and alleviate symptoms like brain fog.

Addressing this deficiency promptly is crucial for maintaining optimal brain health and cognitive function. Alongside supplements, adopting a balanced diet rich in Vitamin B12 sources like meat, fish, eggs, dairy products, and fortified cereals can support brain health and reduce the risk of brain fog.

Once it's confirmed that you have a vitamin B12 deficiency or are at risk for one, you may be advised to take supplements. There are many ways, like tablets, sublingual formulations, and capsules. Dosage will be determined by your unique needs and any underlying medical issues you may have. Always talk to a healthcare professional before supplementing so you can ensure safety and efficacy.

Outside of that, you can increase your consumption through food.

Vitamin B12 Rich Foods

- Beef: Lean cuts provide a moderate amount per serving.
- Clams: These offer a significant portion of the daily recommended intake.

- Eggs: A good source of Vitamin B12, particularly in the yolk.
- Fortified Cereal: Certain cereals are fortified with Vitamin B12, providing a convenient option for vegetarians and vegans.
- Fortified Non-Dairy Milk: Plant-based milk alternatives like soy or almond milk may be fortified with Vitamin B12.
- Fortified Nutritional Yeast: A plant-based source for those following vegetarian or vegan diets.
- Liver and Kidneys: Provides a substantial amount per serving.
- Milk and Dairy Products: Cow's milk, cheese, and yogurt are rich in Vitamin B12.
- Sardines: A good source of Vitamin B12, especially when consumed with the bones.
- Trout and Salmon: Both fish contain Vitamin B12, with salmon offering a higher amount.
- Tuna: Canned tuna is especially high in vitamin B12.

IMPROVING MEMORY FUNCTION WITH DIET: OMEGA-3'S

Omega-3 fatty acids from fish oil are derived from specific fish species, especially those high in DHA (docosahexaenoic acid) and EPA (eicosapentaenoic acid). These fatty acids are widely known for their positive effects on health, particularly when it comes to supporting brain function, cardiovascular health, and general well-being.

The advantages of omega-3 fatty acids come from their makeup, particularly from the higher concentrations of EPA and DHA in comparison to other fatty acids. Both EPA and DHA are essential for preserving good health; EPA has anti-inflammatory properties, while DHA is important for brain development and function (Turner, 2021).

EPA and DHA affect neurotransmitter function, membrane fluidity, and intercellular communication. Improved memory, mood control, and cognitive function are linked to adequate consumption of the two.

The Link Between Fish Oil and Mild Memory Loss

Fish oil rich in omega-3 fatty acids improves cognitive function and lowers the chance of developing the mild memory loss brought on by age. The advantages of EPA and DHA stem from their anti-inflammatory qualities and their function in preserving neural structure and function.

EPA has the potential to reduce symptoms of depression and elevate mood. It helps to control serotonin levels, which are essential for mood management. Women with existing mood disorders or depression may benefit from taking supplements or including fish oil in their diet.

The suggested daily consumption of omega-3 fatty acids varies based on age, health, and specific health goals. However, for overall health, general standards recommend eating at least 250–500 mg of combined EPA and DHA daily.

FOODS HIGH IN OMEGA-3S

- Anchovies: Approximately 1000–2000 mg per 3-ounce serving.
- Caviar: Can provide a substantial amount depending on the type and serving size.
- Chia Seeds: Approximately 4900–5000 mg per ounce.
- Cod Liver Oil: Provides a significant amount, often exceeding daily requirements.
- Flaxseed: Approximately 1800–2000 mg per tablespoon.
- Herring: Approximately 1000–1500 mg per 3-ounce serving.
- Mackerel: Approximately 4500 mg per 3-ounce serving.
- Oysters: Varying levels, with wild-caught varieties being generally higher.
- Salmon: Depending on the variety, 1000–2000 mg per 3-ounce serving.

- Sardines: Approximately 1000–2000 mg per 3-ounce serving.
- Soybeans: Approximately 1000 mg per 3-ounce serving.
- Walnuts: Approximately 2500 mg per ounce.

Other foods and fortified products may also contain Omega-3s, but the amounts can vary widely based on fortification levels. Incorporating a variety of these Omega-3-rich foods into your diet can help you meet daily requirements and support your general health.

Being aware of the subtle changes in memory that occur during menopause enables us to move through this stage with clarity and confidence. It is better to take proactive measures to support cognitive health by understanding the differences between common brain fog and more serious cognitive loss, appreciating the impact of Vitamin B12 insufficiency, and embracing the benefits of Omega-3 fatty acids. The cornerstones of maintaining good brain health during menopause and beyond include adopting lifestyle changes that support brain function, eating a balanced diet rich in vital nutrients, and getting medical advice when needed. We have laid the groundwork for the next chapter's investigation of holistic approaches to health, which includes weight-management techniques.

WEIGHT GAIN

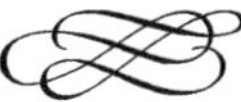

Did you know that 95% of women will experience their final period between the ages of 44 and 56? This highlights the universal yet unique journey of menopause that we undergo (Mahmud, 2023).

WEIGHT GAIN AND MENOPAUSE

The interesting and somewhat frustrating thing about menopause is that it can have an impact on body composition and weight. Hormonal fluctuations are a major factor. Fat tends to shift from the thighs and hips to the tummy as estrogen levels drop. This results in the transition from a pear-shaped physique to an apple one, where most of the weight is concentrated in the waist.

Causes

1. Hormonal Changes: The hormonal shift that comes with menopause can lead to increased fat storage, especially around the abdomen.

2. Lifestyle Factors: Changes in diet, physical activity levels, and stress management can also contribute to weight gain. As we age, we may become less active or experience changes in eating habits, which can impact weight.
3. Decreasing Metabolism: Metabolism naturally slows down with age, leading to fewer calories burned at rest. This makes it easier to gain weight, especially if our dietary habits are not adjusted accordingly.

Impact on Health

Menopausal weight gain is more than just an aesthetic issue. The transition to an apple-shaped body puts us at risk of developing conditions like metabolic syndrome, diabetes, and cardiovascular disease. Insulin resistance and inflammation are two conditions that are exacerbated by excess abdominal fat.

The average weight gain is around 5 pounds, but all our experiences are different. Some of us may not see noticeable changes, while others may gain more than 5 pounds. Weight distribution is influenced by genetics, general health, and lifestyle choices.

WEIGHT MANAGEMENT DURING MENOPAUSE

For effective weight management, we should adopt healthy lifestyle habits, like:

- Balanced Diet: Increase intake of nutrient-dense foods like fruits, vegetables, whole grains, lean proteins, and healthy fats. Limit processed foods, sugary snacks, and excessive alcohol.
- Regular Exercise: Regular physical activity, like cardio, strength training, and flexibility exercises, makes a huge difference. Aim for at least 150 minutes of moderate-intensity exercise per week.

- Stress Management: Practice stress-relieving techniques like mindfulness, yoga, meditation, or deep breathing exercises. Chronic stress contributes to weight gain and other health issues.
- Medical Monitoring: Regular check-ups with your GP can help you monitor weight, assess overall health, and address any underlying medical conditions contributing to any weight changes.

We can manage weight fluctuations more easily and support our general well-being by taking a holistic approach to health that includes good food, exercise, stress reduction, and routine medical treatment.

USING EXERCISE TO FEEL GREAT

With many advantages for mental and physical health, exercise is an invaluable tool during menopause. Frequent exercise can improve your quality of life, help you maintain a healthy weight, and help you manage your symptoms.

The Benefits of Exercise

- Improved Mental Health: Research has indicated that exercise can help reduce the signs and symptoms of anxiety, depression, and mood swings. It makes your body produce more endorphins, or feel-good hormones, that can improve your mood and lower stress levels.
- Improved Physical Health: Exercise can lower your chances of developing chronic illnesses, help you avoid weight gain, and improve heart health. It also raises energy levels, encourages better sleep, and improves general flexibility and mobility.

How to Use It

Have variety. Incorporate a variety of exercises into your routine to target different muscle groups and keep your workouts engaging. Here are some types of exercises to consider:

- Weight-bearing low-impact exercises: Walking, hiking, dancing, and using elliptical machines provide the benefits of weight-bearing exercise without putting too much strain on your joints.
- Weight or strength training: Resistance training using weights, resistance bands, or bodyweight exercises to strengthen muscles, improve bone density, and maintain a healthy metabolism.
- Non-weight-bearing exercises: Swimming and cycling for cardiovascular fitness and muscle toning without hurting the joints.
- Non-impact exercises: Yoga, Pilates, or tai chi focus on flexibility, balance, and core strength, offering gentle yet effective workouts.
- Make it fun: Choose exercises you enjoy to make exercise a positive and enjoyable part of your routine. Whether it's dancing, taking group fitness classes, or exploring outdoor activities, find what brings you joy and keeps you motivated to continue.

The American Heart Association and other health organizations recommend the following exercise guidelines:

- Moderate-intensity exercise: Aim for at least 150 minutes per week by doing 30 minutes of exercise at least five days a week.
- Vigorous exercise: Aim for 75 minutes per week by exercising for just 15 minutes at least five times a week.

- Strength training: Do strength training exercises at least twice a week, targeting major muscle groups with exercises like squats, lunges, push-ups, and lifting weights.

By following these guidelines and incorporating enjoyable activities into your routine, you can reap the benefits of exercise and look after your mental and physical well-being. Remember to listen to your body, start slowly, and consult a healthcare professional before starting any new exercise program, especially if you have pre-existing health conditions.

WAYS TO EXERCISE (WITHOUT REALIZING IT)

Exercise doesn't have to feel like a chore; it can be fun, and you can weave it seamlessly into your daily life. Here are some ideas for staying active without feeling like you're exercising:

1. Active Meetings at Work: Incorporate movement into meetings by having walking meetings or using standing desks. This will keep you engaged, boost your creativity, and promote physical activity.
2. Cleaning: Turn household chores into a workout by cleaning vigorously. It's a practical way to stay active while maintaining a tidy and clean home.
3. Dancing: Turn up the music and dance around your home, join dance classes, or attend social dance events. It is a fun way to burn calories, improve coordination, and lift your mood.
4. Geocaching: Combine treasure hunting with physical activity by participating in geocaching, a global outdoor scavenger hunt using GPS-enabled devices.
5. Golf: Walk the course instead of using a cart, and enjoy the physical benefits of swinging clubs, walking, and engaging in a social activity.

6. Hiking: Explore nature trails, parks, or scenic areas while enjoying the fresh air and beautiful surroundings. Hiking engages your leg muscles, improves cardiovascular fitness, and gives you a mental boost from being outdoors.
7. Jump Rope: Get a quick cardio workout with a jump rope. It improves cardiovascular fitness, coordination, and agility.
8. Kayaking: Explore waterways and lakes while paddling and strengthening your upper body and core muscles.
9. Rock Climbing: Challenge yourself with indoor or outdoor rock climbing sessions. It builds strength, endurance, and coordination while offering a thrilling adventure.
10. Sex: Enjoy the physical benefits of intimacy, which can burn calories, strengthen muscles, and release endorphins.
11. Skiing or Snowboarding: Embrace winter sports for fun and fitness. Skiing and snowboarding strengthen leg muscles, improve balance, and provide a thrilling outdoor experience.
12. Swimming: Dive into swimming for a full-body workout that's gentle on joints. It improves cardiovascular fitness, muscle tone, and endurance.
13. Walking: Take brisk walks during breaks or after meals. Walking is low-impact, easy to do anywhere, and helps maintain overall fitness and mobility.
14. Yoga: Practice yoga for flexibility, balance, and relaxation. It's beneficial for physical and mental well-being, offering various styles to suit different preferences.

By incorporating these enjoyable activities into your routine, you can stay active, boost your fitness levels, and have fun without realizing you're exercising. Choose activities that align with your interests and lifestyle for long-term sustainability and enjoyment.

EATING RIGHT TO AVOID WEIGHT GAIN

Here are essential tips and strategies for healthy eating during this phase:

- Follow Mediterranean diet guidelines: The Mediterranean diet emphasizes whole grains, fruits, vegetables, lean proteins like fish and poultry, healthy fats from olive oil and nuts, and limited red meat and processed foods. This approach is rich in nutrients, antioxidants, and omega-3 fatty acids, supporting heart health and weight management.
- Consume plenty of protein: Incorporate lean proteins like fish, chicken, legumes, tofu, and nuts into your meals. Protein helps build and repair tissues, supports muscle mass, and promotes feelings of fullness, which can help with weight management.
- Include dairy in your diet: Opt for low-fat or non-fat dairy products like yogurt, milk, and cheese. Dairy provides essential nutrients like calcium and vitamin D, which are important for bone health and can contribute to a balanced diet.
- Eat foods high in soluble fiber: Focus on whole grains like oats, quinoa, brown rice, and whole wheat bread. Soluble fiber helps regulate blood sugar levels, makes you feel full, and supports digestive health.
- Eat fruits and vegetables first: Start meals with a serving of fruits or vegetables to increase fiber intake and fill up on nutrient-dense foods. Include a variety of colorful fruits and vegetables to benefit from different vitamins, minerals, and antioxidants.

Practice Mindful Eating

It is a practice that encourages awareness of food choices, eating habits, and sensations while eating. It involves

- Being present: Focus on the present while eating, savor flavors, textures, and smells.
- Eating slowly: Take time to chew thoroughly and allow your body to register fullness cues to prevent overeating.
- Paying attention to hunger cues: Eat when you're hungry and stop when you're comfortably full. Pay attention to internal cues rather than external ones.
- Avoiding distractions: Minimize distractions like screens or multitasking while eating to fully experience meals and promote mindful eating habits.

What to Avoid

- Excess Salt: Limit salt intake to support heart health and prevent water retention.
- Hidden Sugars: Be mindful of added sugars in processed foods, sugary drinks, and snacks. Opt for naturally sweetened foods, or cut down on sugary treats.
- Limit Caffeine and Alcohol: Reduce caffeine and alcohol consumption, as they can interfere with sleep, hydration, and overall health.
- Avoid or Limit Fried Foods: Opt for healthier cooking methods like baking, grilling, or steaming instead of frying to reduce excess calories and unhealthy fats.

By following these healthy eating tips, practicing mindful eating, and being mindful of food choices, you can navigate menopause with a balanced approach to nutrition, supporting weight management and your overall health.

EMBRACING BODY POSITIVITY

In a culture that is fixated on youth and beauty, menopausal women feel pressured to maintain a certain appearance. The notion that being young and slender equals worth and desirability is promoted by the media and advertising sectors. These industries uphold unattainable beauty standards. The pressure from society to maintain beauty and youth can negatively impact menopausal women's self-perception. Women who feel compelled to live up to these standards may feel inadequate, have low self-esteem, and be dissatisfied with their bodies. This can exacerbate conditions like anxiety and depression and lead to feelings of isolation.

It's important to understand that you are ultimately responsible for how you view aging and attractiveness. Challenging society's expectations and valuing your individual experience are key components of embracing body positivity during menopause. Focus on feeling strong, confident, and healthy in your own skin rather than aiming for unachievable beauty standards.

This kind of body positivity needs you to shift your perspective. Think of the changes in your body as natural changes, as opposed to failures. This is a life-changing stage that should offer insight, life experience, and a more profound comprehension of oneself. Honor the process and put more emphasis on general well-being than looks.

How You Can Foster Body Positivity

- Put Health First: Shift the focus from weight loss to overall health and well-being. Engage in activities that nourish your body, mind, and soul.
- Challenge Negative Thoughts: Challenge negative thoughts about aging and body image. Replace critical thoughts with positive affirmations that celebrate your strengths, resilience, and unique beauty.
- Surround Yourself With Positivity: Surround yourself with supportive and positive influences. Look for communities, friends, and resources that promote body positivity and self-acceptance.

- Engage in Self-Care: Prioritize self-care activities that make you feel good about yourself. Self-care is essential for nurturing a positive body image.
- Practice Self-Compassion: Be kind to yourself. Treat yourself with the same kindness and understanding you would other people.

Throughout menopause, you can develop a more loving and understanding relationship with your body by adopting a body-positive mindset. Your value and worth go well beyond how you look, and the secret to prospering at this life-changing stage is to embrace your journey with self-love and confidence. Next, we will explore alternative medicine approaches to managing menopause symptoms.

PART III
NATURAL REMEDIES AND RESOURCES

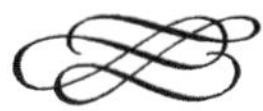

ALTERNATIVE MEDICINE

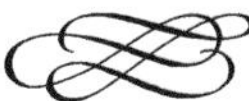

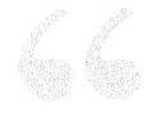

Menopause. A pause while you reconsider men.

— MARGARET ATWOOD

ACUPUNCTURE

In the holistic healthcare world, acupuncture stands out as a centuries-old practice deeply rooted in traditional Chinese medicine. It is the strategic placement of fine needles at specific points on the body, aiming to stimulate energy flow along pathways called meridians. This stimulation is believed to restore balance to the body's energy and promote healing.

The exact science behind it is multifaceted and still under scientific investigation. One proposed explanation is its impact on the nervous system. Inserting needles triggers nerve endings, prompting the release of biochemicals like endorphins, which are the body's natural painkillers. This process can modulate pain perception and may also affect neurotransmitter levels, influencing mood and stress responses.

For menopausal women, acupuncture is a holistic approach to alleviating a spectrum of symptoms.

Research and anecdotal evidence suggest that acupuncture may provide relief for these symptoms by regulating hormonal balance, improving circulation, and enhancing relaxation. It's important that you seek a qualified practitioner or healthcare professional who is experienced in women's health and menopausal care. A tailored treatment plan may involve regular acupuncture sessions, dietary and lifestyle changes, herbal supplements, and other complementary therapies to address your unique needs (Olesinski, 2024).

Menopausal symptoms that acupuncture can help to relieve:

- hot flashes
- night sweats
- pain
- mood swings
- anxiety
- insomnia
- fatigue
- vaginal dryness

COGNITIVE BEHAVIORAL THERAPY

The goal of cognitive behavioral therapy, or CBT, is to recognize and change harmful thought processes and behavior patterns that underlie emotional suffering and mental health problems. It highlights the relationship between ideas, emotions, and actions with the goal of swapping out harmful beliefs for more adaptive and pleasant ones.

By targeting the cognitive and behavioral processes that lead to distress and discomfort during this transition, CBT has shown efficacy in helping women manage their symptoms.

How Does It Work?

CBT targets the following:

- Physical Symptoms, i.e., hot flashes, mood swings, and insomnia.
- Thoughts: Negative thoughts and beliefs about aging and symptom severity.
- Feelings: Emotional responses like anxiety, frustration, or sadness related to symptoms.
- Behavior: Coping behaviors or avoidance strategies that may exacerbate symptoms or impact daily functioning.

CBT as a Treatment for Menopause

Studies back up CBT's efficacy in lowering menopause-related symptoms and general quality of life. Research has indicated that symptom intensity and psychological well-being can be improved by using CBT techniques customized for menopausal women (Trudel-Fitzgerald et al., 2019).

1. Cognitive Restructuring: Identify and challenge negative thoughts and beliefs about menopause and replace them with more balanced and positive ones.
2. Behavioral Activation: Engage in activities that promote a sense of accomplishment, pleasure, and relaxation, helping to counteract feelings of lethargy or fatigue.
3. Mindfulness Techniques: Practice mindfulness and relaxation exercises to increase awareness of the moment, reduce stress, and promote emotional regulation.

BREATHING EXERCISES

Breathing exercises are often overlooked, but they actually work really well for managing menopausal symptoms. The link between breathwork and healing lies in the mind and body connection. Here's how breathwork can help alleviate your symptoms:

- Cooling for the mind and body: Certain techniques, like the cooling breath, can help regulate body temperature and mitigate hot flashes.
- Presence and mindfulness: Breath-focused practices cultivate mindfulness and presence, helping us navigate these changes with greater awareness and acceptance, reducing reactivity to symptoms and enhancing emotional resilience.
- Relieves an anxious mind: Controlled breathing techniques can soothe an anxious mind, improve focus, and enhance mental clarity, which can be particularly beneficial during emotional fluctuations.
- Stillness: Incorporating breathwork into a daily routine creates moments of stillness and inner calm, providing a sanctuary from the hustle and bustle of life and fostering a deeper connection with oneself.
- Stress reduction: Menopause can bring about heightened stress levels due to hormonal fluctuations and associated symptoms. Breathwork triggers the relaxation response, reducing stress hormones like cortisol and promoting a sense of calm and well-being.

Let's delve into specific breathwork techniques that you can practice at home to address your symptoms:

Bumble Bee Breath

Step-By-Step Instructions

1. Close your eyes and take a deep breath in.
2. As you exhale, gently press your fingers against your ears to partially close them; this creates a humming sound like that of a bumblebee.

3. Continue for several breaths, focusing on the soothing vibration and sound.

Helps With

- It is effective for calming the mind, reducing stress, and promoting relaxation. It can be helpful when you experience mood swings or insomnia.

Straw Breath

Step-By-Step Instructions

1. Inhale gently through a narrow imaginary straw or a real one held between your lips, allowing your breath to be slow and controlled.
2. Exhale smoothly through the nose or mouth. Repeat several times.

Helps With

- It calms the nervous system, reducing anxiety and promoting a sense of peace. You can use it whenever you feel overwhelmed, anxious, or in need of a moment of peace and quiet.

The Hot Flash Wave

Step-By-Step Instructions

1. Sit comfortably with your spine erect.
2. Take a slow, deep breath through your nose, to expand your belly and rib cage.
3. Hold it for a moment, then exhale slowly through pursed lips, like you are blowing out a candle.

4. Repeat this cycle for 5–10 breaths.

Helps With

- This technique helps manage hot flashes by promoting relaxation and a sense of cooling in the body. Use it when you feel a hot flash coming on or as a preventive measure.

YOGA

Yoga is good for managing both physical and emotional changes. Here's why incorporating it into your routine can be transformative:

- Balance moods and emotions: The mind-body connection helps to balance emotions and enhance mental clarity, which should reduce mood swings and promote emotional stability.
- Boost slow metabolism: Yoga can stimulate metabolism through movement and targeted poses, supporting weight management and overall vitality.
- Reduce stress: Yoga practices, like deep breathing and mindfulness, can help reduce stress hormones like cortisol, promoting a sense of calm.
- Release physical stress and tension: Menopause can bring about physical discomfort and tension in the body. Yoga poses and stretches target areas of tension, promote flexibility, and release tight muscles.
- Restore energy: Yoga practices, like gentle flows and restorative poses, can help replenish your energy levels and fight fatigue.
- Strengthen muscles and build bone density: Weight-bearing yoga poses and strength-building sequences can help maintain muscle mass and bone density.

Yoga is a practice that evolves with age, offering tailored benefits to support our well-being as we grow older. It promotes flexibility, balance, and strength, which are essential for maintaining mobility and preventing injuries. It also cultivates mindfulness and resilience, which makes you more adaptable to life's changes and challenges.

Here are some poses you can try to alleviate your symptoms:

Cat/Cow Pose (*Marjaryasana/Bitilasana*)

Instructions

1. Start on your hands and knees, aligning your wrists under your shoulders and your knees under your hips.
2. Inhale, arch your back, then lift your head and tailbone (Cow Pose).
3. Exhale, round your spine, tuck your chin into your chest and tuck your tailbone (Cat Pose).
4. Repeat, and sync your breath with your movement.

Benefits

Helps improve spinal flexibility, relieves tension in the back and neck, massages internal organs, and promotes a healthy spine.

Fan Posture (*Viparita Karani*)

Instructions

1. Lie on your back near a wall, with your hips touching the wall and legs extended upward along the wall.
2. Put your arms in a comfortable position, either on your sides or resting on your belly.
3. Relax and breathe deeply, allowing your body to be supported by the wall.

Benefits

This posture is a restorative inversion that promotes relaxation, relieves swelling in the legs and feet, improves circulation, and calms your nervous system.

Forward-Facing Hero Pose (*Ardha Ustrasana*)

Instructions

1. Kneel on the mat with your knees hip-width apart.
2. Put your hands on your lower back for support.
3. Inhale, lift your chest, and gently arch backward, keeping your hips aligned over your knees.
4. Hold your pose for a few breaths, then return to a neutral position.

Benefits

This pose stretches the front of your body, opens up the chest and shoulders, strengthens back muscles, and improves spinal flexibility.

Lunge Pose (*Anjaneyasana*)

Instructions

1. From a standing position, step one foot back into a lunge, keeping your front knee directly over your ankle.
2. Lower your back knee to the mat, or keep it lifted for a deeper stretch.
3. Raise your arms over your head or place your hands on your front thigh.
4. Hold the pose and breathe deeply for several breaths, then switch sides.

Benefits

This pose stretches the hips, thighs, and groin. It also improves balance, strengthens the legs, and opens the chest and shoulders.

Sphinx Pose (*Salamba Bhujangasana*)

Instructions

1. Lie on your tummy with your legs extended and forearms on the ground, elbows under your shoulders.
2. Press your forearms into the mat, lift your chest and head, and lengthen your spine.
3. Keep your shoulders relaxed and look forward while breathing deeply.

Benefits

This pose gently stretches the spine, opens your chest and shoulders, strengthens the back muscles, and improves your posture.

If you practice yoga often enough, you will age gracefully, experience relief from your symptoms, and improve your well-being. Always listen to your body and make changes to the poses to suit your comfort level.

HYPNOSIS

By inducing a state of profound relaxation and heightened concentration, hypnosis acts as a treatment that makes it easier for people to tap into their subconscious minds. In order to promote constructive changes in attitudes, feelings, and actions, it makes use of suggestion, focused attention, and guided imagery.

Due to its potential advantages in fostering relaxation, lowering stress, introducing coping mechanisms, and easing symptoms, some women may resort to hypnosis.

What Are the Benefits?

- Relaxation: An induced state of relaxation can help reduce tension, anxiety, and stress levels.
- Symptom Reduction: Hypnosis has been associated with decreased frequency and intensity of hot flashes, improved sleep quality, and enhanced emotional well-being.

Hypnosis has been shown in numerous studies to be effective in treating menopausal symptoms. Studies have shown that menopausal women's quality of life and the severity of their symptoms can be improved with hypnotherapy (Sutton, 2021).

Hypnotherapy Techniques You Can Use

Cool Imagery

Instructions:

1. Find a quiet and comfortable space to sit or lie down.
2. Close your eyes and take slow, deep breaths to relax.
3. Visualize a serene and cool environment, like a snowy landscape or a refreshing ocean breeze.
4. Imagine and focus on the sensations of coolness and calmness spreading throughout your body.
5. Keep yourself in this imagery for several minutes, breathing deeply and enjoying the sense of relaxation and relief.

Flash Control Dial

Instructions:

1. Close your eyes and imagine a control dial in front of you, labeled with the specific symptom you want to address.
2. Visualize turning the dial down gradually, decreasing the intensity and frequency of the symptom.

3. As you turn the dial, imagine cooler sensations and a sense of calm spreading through your body.
4. Repeat this until you feel a sense of relief and control over the symptom.

Your Future Self

Instructions:

1. Imagine yourself in the future, free from your symptoms and feeling vibrant and healthy.
2. Picture yourself doing all the activities you enjoy while feeling confident and empowered.
3. Focus on the positive emotions and sensations associated with this self-image.
4. Use affirmations or positive statements to reinforce the vision so you can build optimism about your well-being.

You could benefit from practicing hypnosis techniques regularly. Integrating them into your self-care regimen can help you manage your symptoms, encourage relaxation, and improve your general well-being.

Menopause brings a myriad of challenges that affect both physical and emotional well-being. By incorporating holistic practices like acupuncture, cognitive behavioral therapy, breathwork, yoga, and hypnosis into your routine, you can alleviate many symptoms. These methods not only promote relaxation and balance but also empower you to manage this transition with more ease and resilience. As you try these approaches, remember the importance of tailoring them to your unique needs and getting guidance from qualified practitioners. Moving forward, we will delve into supplements and natural medicine. We will explore various vitamins, minerals, and herbal remedies that can further support your health and well-being during this time. By understanding the role of natural medicine, you can create a comprehensive and personalized plan to navigate menopause with confidence and vitality.

SUPPLEMENTS AND NATURAL MEDICINE

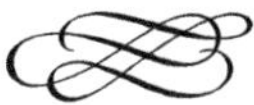

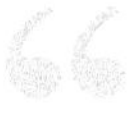

> *Fifty was a shock, because it was the end of the center period of life. But once I got over that, 60 was great. Seventy was great. And I loved, I seriously loved aging.*
>
> — YOKO ONO

BLACK COHOSH

Black cohosh is a perennial herb native to North America, historically used by Native American tribes for medicinal purposes. It grows in woodland areas and is known for its tall, white flower spikes. The root is the part most commonly used in herbal medicine. It's gaining a lot of popularity as a natural symptom reliever because of its effectiveness in lessening the frequency and intensity of menopausal symptoms. It has the ability to boost estrogen levels, but the process is still being studied (*Black Cohosh: Uses, Side Effects, Interactions, Dosage, and Warning*, 2019).

It helps with

- Hot flashes and night sweats: It is believed to act on the hypothalamus, the part of the brain that regulates body temperature.
- Mood swings and emotional well-being: By influencing serotonin receptors, it can help stabilize mood and reduce anxiety and the depressive symptoms that often accompany menopause.
- Vaginal dryness: The potential estrogenic effects may also help alleviate vaginal dryness.

How to Use It

Black Cohosh comes in many forms: capsules, tablets, liquid extracts, and teas. You can manage your symptoms by using a standardized extract of the herb.

- Capsules/Tablets: These are the most convenient. The typical dosage ranges from 20 to 80 mg per day. They contain 1 mg of triterpene and glycosides, which are the active compounds in black cohosh.
- Liquid Extracts: These can be mixed with water or juice. The recommendation is 2 to 4 ml of a 1:5 ratio tincture taken three times daily.
- Teas: These are less common, but tea can be made by steeping 1 to 2 grams of dried root in boiling water for 10 to 15 minutes. However, this method may not provide a consistent dosage of the active ingredients.

Potential Side Effects

Although black cohosh is generally regarded as safe for short-term use (up to six months), some people may experience side effects. Potential side effects include:

1. Gastrointestinal distress: Nausea, stomach cramps, and diarrhea.
2. Headaches.
3. Dizziness or lightheadedness.
4. Liver issues: There have been rare reports of liver damage, so if you have a liver condition, practice caution and consult a healthcare professional before use.

Standard Dosage

- Capsules/Tablets: 20 to 80 mg daily, divided into two doses if needed.
- Liquid Extracts: 2 to 4 ml, taken up to three times per day.
- Tea: One cup made with 1 to 2 grams of dried root once or twice per day.

It's important to follow the dosage instructions laid out by the manufacturer or a healthcare professional because excessive use can increase the risk of side effects.

EVENING PRIMROSE OIL

Evening primrose oil (EPO) is a natural supplement derived from the seeds of the evening primrose plant, a wildflower native to North America. It produces bright yellow flowers that bloom in the evening, hence the name. The oil extracted from its seeds is rich in gamma-linolenic acid (GLA), an omega-6 fatty acid known for its anti-inflammatory properties and health benefits.

Benefits

A variety of symptoms can be relieved using evening primrose oil because of its special composition and qualities. Benefits include:

1. Hot Flashes: The GLA in evening primrose oil can influence prostaglandin synthesis, which plays a role in temperature regulation.
2. Mood Swings and Emotional Well-Being: The anti-inflammatory properties of GLA may help stabilize mood and reduce the irritability and depression associated with hormonal fluctuations.
3. Breast Pain (Mastalgia): EPO has been shown to alleviate breast pain by reducing inflammation and balancing hormone levels (*Evening Primrose Oil*, n.d.).
4. Skin Health: The essential fatty acids in EPO help maintain skin moisture and improve overall skin health.

Potential Side Effects

While it is generally considered safe for most people, it can cause side effects in some. These may include:

- Gastrointestinal Issues: Nausea, stomach pain, and diarrhea.
- Headaches.
- Allergic Reactions: EPO can seldom cause allergic reactions, including rash, swelling, and difficulty breathing.
- Blood Thinning: EPO may have a mild blood-thinning effect, so it should be used with caution if you are taking anticoagulant medications.

How to Take It

EPO is available in capsules, liquid extracts, and topical applications. The appropriate dosage varies based on the symptoms and individual needs.

- Capsules: These are the most common form of supplement. The typical dosage ranges from 500 mg to 1,000 mg, taken

one to three times daily. Each capsule usually contains a standardized amount of GLA.
- Liquid Extracts: These can be mixed with food or drinks. The recommended dosage is generally similar to that of capsules, but it is advised that you follow the manufacturer's instructions or a healthcare provider's guidance.
- Topical Applications: For skin-related issues, you can apply EPO directly to the skin. It is particularly useful for conditions like eczema or dry skin.

Standard Dosage

For managing menopausal symptoms, a common dosage recommendation is 500 mg to 1,000 mg one to three times daily, as this dosage provides a sufficient amount of GLA.

It's important to start with a lower dose and gradually increase it to assess tolerance and avoid potential side effects. Consult with a healthcare professional, especially if you are on other medication or have underlying health issues.

SOY

Soy is a versatile legume native to East Asia. It is known for its high protein content and health benefits. It is taken from the soybean (*Glycine max*) and is consumed in many forms, including tofu, tempeh, soy milk, and soy protein isolates. It is rich in isoflavones, plant compounds that mimic the activity of estrogen in the body, making it great for managing menopausal symptoms.

Benefits

The isoflavones found in soy, primarily genistein and daidzein, are phytoestrogens. These are plant-derived compounds that can promote estrogen-like effects in the body. This makes soy an effective natural remedy for several symptoms:

- Hot Flashes: Soy isoflavones can bind to estrogen receptors, helping to regulate temperature and reduce the frequency and severity of hot flashes.
- Night Sweats: Similar to its effect on hot flashes, soy can help alleviate night sweats, improving sleep quality and overall comfort.
- Bone Health: Soy isoflavones can help mitigate menopause's effect on bone density by promoting bone health and reducing the risk of fractures.
- Mood Stability: Soy isoflavones have been shown to have a stabilizing effect on mood, helping to reduce emotional disturbances.
- Weight Management: Soy is a low-calorie, high-protein food that can help with weight management by promoting satiety and preserving lean muscle mass.

Potential Side Effects

While soy is generally safe for most people, it can cause side effects in some, especially when consumed in large amounts:

- Digestive Issues: Soy can cause mild gastrointestinal discomfort, like bloating, gas, or constipation.
- Allergic Reactions: Symptoms of Soy allergies include hives, itching, and, in severe cases, anaphylaxis.
- Hormonal Effects: Given its estrogen-like activity, excessive soy consumption might interfere with thyroid function or affect hormonal balance, particularly in women with thyroid disorders or hormone-sensitive conditions.

How to Take It

Soy can be incorporated into your diet in many forms, which makes it flexible for different preferences and dietary needs. These are some common ways to consume soy:

- Edamame: Young, green soybeans that are steamed or boiled. They can be a nutritious snack or can be added to salads for extra protein and fiber.
- Soy Milk: A plant-based milk made from soybeans. It is mostly used in smoothies, cereals, and baking. It is a good source of protein, calcium (when fortified), and vitamin D.
- Soy Protein Isolate: A very refined form of soy protein, mostly used in protein powders and supplements. It is an excellent source of protein, providing all the essential amino acids needed by your body.
- Tempeh: A fermented soy product that is firm and has a nutty flavor. It can be sliced, marinated, and cooked in many ways, making it a versatile protein source for meals.
- Tofu: Made from coagulated soy milk, it is a versatile ingredient. It can be grilled, stir-fried, or added to soups and salads. Tofu comes in different textures, from silken to extra-firm, so it is suitable for a wide range of recipes.

Dosage

The amount of soy needed to achieve its health benefits can vary, but general guidelines suggest:

- For Menopausal Symptoms: 40–80 mg of soy isoflavones per day. This can be achieved through dietary sources or supplements.
- Dietary Sources: 1–2 servings of soy-based foods daily can provide the necessary isoflavones.

Soy, with its rich content of isoflavones, offers a natural and effective way to manage menopausal symptoms. Its additional benefits for heart health, bone health, and cancer prevention make it a valuable addition to your diet. It's important to consume it in moderation and be aware of the potential side effects.

GINSENG

Ginseng is a well-known herb, popular for its medicinal properties. It has been used for centuries in traditional Chinese medicine and is revered for its ability to enhance vitality, boost energy, and improve overall well-being. There are several varieties, but Asian ginseng (*Panax ginseng*) and American ginseng (*Panax quinquefolius*) are the most commonly used.

The root of the ginseng plant is the part used for its medicinal properties. Asian ginseng is primarily found in Korea, China, and parts of Russia, while American ginseng is native to the forests of North America, particularly the United States and Canada. The roots are harvested after several years of growth, with older roots considered more potent.

Benefits

Ginseng has shown promise in alleviating symptoms due to its adaptogenic properties, which help the body adapt to stress and maintain homeostasis. The key benefits include:

- Hot Flashes and Night Sweats: Ginseng can help reduce the frequency and intensity of hot flashes and night sweats. Red ginseng, in particular, can be effective in alleviating these common symptoms.
- Mood and Cognitive Function: Ginseng has the potential to enhance mood and cognitive function. It can help with mood

swings, depression, and anxiety. Its neuroprotective effects support brain health and improve mental clarity.
- Fatigue and Energy Levels: Ginseng is well-known for its ability to combat fatigue and boost energy levels. This is beneficial for women experiencing chronic tiredness and lack of energy.

Potential Side Effects

- Ginseng is generally considered safe for most people, but it can cause side effects in some, especially when taken in large doses or for extended periods:
- Allergic Reactions: Although rare, allergic reactions can occur, presenting symptoms like hives, itching, or difficulty breathing.
- Digestive Issues: Ginseng can cause mild gastrointestinal issues like nausea, diarrhea, or stomach cramps.
- Headaches: Some people may experience headaches or dizziness when taking ginseng.
- Insomnia: Due to its stimulating properties, ginseng can cause insomnia or sleep disturbances if taken too close to bedtime.

Dosage

Ginseng can be consumed in many forms, like capsules, tablets, teas, extracts, and powders. How you consume it depends on personal preference and the specific type of product available to you.

- Capsules/Tablets: Convenient and easy to dose.
- Tea: Ginseng root can be brewed into tea.
- Extracts/Tinctures: Liquid extracts are highly concentrated and can be added to water or other beverages.
- Powders: Ginseng powder can be mixed into smoothies, juices, or food.

- For Menopausal Symptoms: 200–400 mg of standardized extract per day, divided into two doses. Start with a lower dose, then gradually increase.

Consult a healthcare provider before you start consuming ginseng, especially if you have underlying health conditions or are taking other medications.

RED CLOVER

Red clover (*Trifolium pratense*) is a perennial herbaceous plant in the legume family. It has distinctive red or purplish flowers and is native to Europe, Western Asia, and northwest Africa, but has also been naturalized in North America. It has been used in traditional medicine practices for various ailments because of its rich composition of bioactive compounds.

Benefits

Red clover has isoflavones, plant-based compounds that mimic estrogen in the body. These isoflavones, including biochanin A, daidzein, genistein, and formononetin, can help alleviate various symptoms by balancing hormone levels. The primary benefits of red clover include:

- Hot Flashes and Night Sweats: Red clover's isoflavones can reduce the frequency and severity of hot flashes and night sweats.
- Cardiovascular Health: Isoflavones can improve blood vessel health and reduce the risk of cardiovascular diseases, which is a concern for postmenopausal women.
- Bone Health: Red clover can support bone density and reduce the risk of osteoporosis, which is a common issue after menopause.

Beyond symptoms, red clover offers other health benefits, including:

- Skin Health: Red clover has been used topically to treat skin conditions like eczema and psoriasis.
- Anti-Inflammatory Effects: Its anti-inflammatory properties can help with conditions like arthritis.

Potential Side Effects

Red clover is generally considered safe for most people when taken in appropriate doses; however, it can cause some side effects, like

- mild nausea
- headaches
- skin rashes
- In rare cases, it may interfere with hormone-sensitive conditions and anticoagulant medications.

Dosage

Red clover can be consumed in many forms, each with specific dosage recommendations:

- Dried herb: Can be used to make teas or infusions. A typical dose is 1–2 teaspoons per cup of boiling water, steeped for 10–15 minutes.
- Powdered herb: Can be added to smoothies, juices, or other foods. The dosage typically ranges from 1 to 2 grams per day.
- Tincture: A concentrated liquid extract. The usual dose is 30–60 drops three times per day.
- Fluid extract: More concentrated than tinctures. The typical dose is 2–4 ml, three times per day.
- Standardized red clover isoflavone extracts: These supplements contain a standardized amount of isoflavones.

Dosage varies, but a common range is 40–80 mg of isoflavones per day.
- Topical treatments: Creams or ointments containing red clover extracts can be applied directly to the skin for conditions like eczema or psoriasis.

WHO SHOULD AVOID IT?

Some women should avoid red clover, including:

- Women with hormone-sensitive conditions: Women with breast cancer, uterine cancer, ovarian cancer, endometriosis, or uterine fibroids should avoid red clover as it may exacerbate these conditions.
- Women on anticoagulant medications: Red clover can interfere with blood-thinning medications, increasing the risk of bleeding.

By understanding the benefits and potential risks, you can make informed decisions about incorporating this herbal remedy into your management plan.

DONG QUAI

Dong Quai, often referred to as the female ginseng, is a traditional herbal remedy with a rich history in Chinese medicine. It is known for its potential to alleviate menopausal symptoms. It has become increasingly popular in the West for its health benefits, particularly for women undergoing the hormonal changes of menopause.

Dong Quai (*Angelica sinensis*) is a perennial plant native to the high-altitude regions of China, Japan, and Korea. It belongs to the same botanical family as carrots and celery, the *Apiaceae* family. Its roots are harvested and used for medicinal purposes. It thrives in the cool, damp climates of East Asia. It has been a staple in Chinese herbal medicine and is often used in combination with other herbs to balance female hormones and treat various conditions related to women's health.

Benefits

Dong Quai is popular for its potential to alleviate several symptoms:

- Hormonal Balance: Dong Quai contains phytoestrogens, which are plant-based compounds that mimic the effects of estrogen in the body. This makes it useful for managing symptoms caused by the decline in estrogen levels during menopause.
- Menstrual Health: Although it's known for its menopausal benefits, Dong Quai has traditionally been used to regulate menstrual cycles and alleviate menstrual cramps. For women transitioning into menopause, this can help them manage their irregular periods.
- Mood Stabilization: Dong Quai's balancing effects on hormones may help to stabilize mood and improve emotional well-being.
- Bone Health: The estrogen-like effects of Dong Quai can also contribute to maintaining bone density and reducing the risk of osteoporosis, which is a concern for many postmenopausal women.

Potential Side Effects

While Dong Quai is generally considered safe when used appropriately, it can cause side effects in some. Potential side effects include:

- Photosensitivity: Increased sensitivity to sunlight leads to a higher risk of sunburn.

- Bleeding Disorders: Due to its blood-thinning properties, Dong Quai should be used with caution if you have a bleeding disorder or are taking anticoagulant medications.
- Digestive Issues: Some people may experience gastrointestinal symptoms like nausea, diarrhea, or stomach cramps.

Always consult a healthcare provider before starting Dong Quai, especially if you have underlying health conditions or are taking other medications.

Dosage

Dong Quai is available in many forms, allowing for flexible use depending on your preferences and needs. Here are the common forms and dosage recommendations:

Capsules or Tablets

Dosage: 500-600 mg, taken one to three times daily. It is important to follow the dosage instructions on the product label or as advised by a healthcare professional.

Tinctures

Dosage: Tinctures are concentrated liquid extracts. The usual recommendation is 1–2 ml, taken two to three times daily. They can be added to water or juice for easier consumption.

Powder

Dosage: Dong Quai powder can be mixed into teas, smoothies, or other beverages. The standard dosage is about 1/4 to 1/2 teaspoon per serving, taken one to three times daily.

Things to Consider

- Start Slow: Start with a lower dose and gradually increase it to monitor how your body responds.

- Be consistent: Regular, consistent use is key. This way, you can experience the benefits of Dong Quai. It may take several weeks to notice significant improvements.
- Consult: Always consult a healthcare professional before starting any new supplement regimen.

Besides its effectiveness in alleviating menopausal symptoms, Dong Quai's anti-inflammatory and cardiovascular benefits further enhance its appeal. However, like any supplement, use it with caution and under the guidance of a healthcare professional to ensure safety and effectiveness.

VALERIAN

Valerian is a herb that has been used for centuries to treat a range of ailments, particularly related to sleep and anxiety. It is known for its sedative properties and is derived from the root of the *Valeriana officinalis* plant. It is a natural remedy for promoting relaxation and improving sleep quality.

Valerian is a perennial flowering plant native to Europe and parts of Asia. It is also grown in North America. It produces sweetly scented pink or white flowers, but it is the root that contains the compounds responsible for its medicinal properties. Valerian root is harvested and dried to be used in various forms, including teas, capsules, tablets, and tinctures.

Benefits

Valerian helps to alleviate several common symptoms:

- Sleep Disorders: Valerian is well-known for its sedative effects, which can help improve sleep quality and lessen the time it takes to fall asleep.

- Anxiety and Mood Swings: Valerian has anxiolytic properties that help calm the nervous system, which can reduce feelings of anxiety and stress. This leads to better moods and emotional stability.
- Hot Flashes and Night Sweats: Valerian's calming effects on the nervous system can provide relief from these disruptive symptoms, resulting in better sleep and overall comfort.

Potential Side Effects

Valerian is generally safe for most people when taken as directed, but it can cause side effects in some:

- Drowsiness: Due to its sedative effects, it can cause drowsiness, especially if taken during the day.
- Dizziness: Some women may experience dizziness or lightheadedness.
- Digestive Issues: Nausea, stomach cramps, and diarrhea are possible side effects, especially when taken in large doses.
- Headaches: Although rare, it can cause headaches in some.

Dosage

Valerian can be consumed in different forms, making it a versatile option if you are looking to incorporate it into your routine. The most common forms include capsules, tablets, teas, and tinctures.

- Capsules/Tablets: These are convenient and provide a precise dosage.
- Tea: Tea can be made by steeping 2–3 grams of dried root in hot water for 10–15 minutes.
- Tinctures: Liquid extracts are concentrated and can be added to water or other beverages.
- For Sleep Disorders: 300–600 mg of valerian root extract, taken 30 minutes to two hours before bedtime. Always follow

the dosage instructions on the product label or as recommended by a healthcare professional.

- For Anxiety and Stress: A lower dose of 150–300 mg, taken one to three times daily. Start with a lower dose and then adjust as needed.

Always consult a healthcare provider before starting valerian, especially if you have underlying health conditions or are taking other medications. Valerian should not be combined with other sedative medications or alcohol because of the risk of excessive drowsiness.

ST JOHN'S WORT

St. John's Wort is a versatile herb used in traditional medicine. It helps to alleviate some menopausal symptoms. It is known for its antidepressant properties and is used to treat mild to moderate depression and other mood disorders. This makes it perfect for menopausal women who may be experiencing psychological challenges.

It is a flowering plant native to Europe but is now found in many temperate regions worldwide, including North America, Asia, and Australia. It gets its name from St. John the Baptist because it typically blooms around his feast day on June 24th. Its bright yellow flowers have been used for medicinal purposes for over 2,000 years (*St. John's Wort: Uses, Side Effects, Interactions, Dosage, and Warning,* 2017).

It was originally a remedy for wounds, burns, and other ailments. Today, it is primarily known for its mental health benefits, like managing depression and anxiety.

Benefits

St. John's Wort addresses several common symptoms:

- Mood Disorders: St. John's Wort is renowned for its antidepressant effects, which can help stabilize mood and alleviate feelings of sadness and anxiety. Studies have shown that it can be as effective as some prescription antidepressants in treating mild to moderate depression without the associated side effects (Fallis, 2024).

- Hot Flashes: Its mood-enhancing properties can indirectly improve overall well-being, making it easier to cope with hot flashes and night sweats.
- Sleep Disorders: By alleviating anxiety and depression, St. John's Wort can improve sleep quality, helping you achieve more restful and uninterrupted sleep.

Potential Side Effects

St. John's Wort is generally safe for most people when taken at recommended doses; however, it can cause side effects and interact with other medications. Potential side effects include:

- Gastrointestinal Issues: Nausea, diarrhea, and stomach cramps.
- Dizziness and Fatigue: Some women may experience dizziness, fatigue, or restlessness.
- Photosensitivity: St. John's Wort can increase sensitivity to sunlight, leading to a higher risk of sunburn or skin rash. Use sunscreen and wear protective clothing when spending time outdoors.
- Drug Interactions: This herb can interact with several medications, like antidepressants, birth control pills, blood thinners, and certain chemotherapy drugs. These interactions can reduce the effectiveness of medications or increase the risk of side effects. Always consult with a healthcare professional before starting St. John's Wort, especially if you are on other medication.

Dosage

St. John's Wort is available in many forms, including capsules, tablets, teas, and liquid extracts. The form you choose may depend on personal preference and the health issue you are addressing.

- Capsules/Tablets: These are convenient and provide a precise dosage. Go for standardized extracts containing 0.3% hypericin, which is the active compound.
- Tea: Tea can be made by steeping 1–2 teaspoons of dried herb in hot water for 10–15 minutes. It is less potent than standardized extracts but can still offer benefits.
- Liquid Extracts: These are concentrated and can be added to water or other beverages. Follow the dosage instructions provided by the manufacturer.
- For Mood Disorders: 300 mg of extract, taken three times daily. This dosage can be adjusted based on your response and under the guidance of a healthcare professional.
- For Menopausal Symptoms: A similar dosage of 300 mg, taken two to three times daily, can help manage mood swings and hot flashes. It may take several weeks of consistent use to notice improvements.

Start with a lower dose and gradually increase to minimize potential side effects. Regular monitoring and consultation with a healthcare professional is essential, especially if you are combining it with other treatments.

As you navigate through this transformative period, remember that you have a multitude of natural remedies at your disposal. Black cohosh, evening primrose oil, soy, ginseng, red clover, and Dong Quai each offer unique benefits to help alleviate the physical and emotional symptoms associated with this stage of life. By understanding their uses, benefits, potential side effects, and proper dosages, you can make informed decisions about incorporating them into your health regimen.

Menopause is not an end but rather a new beginning, a time to embrace change and focus on self-care. With the right approach, you can manage symptoms effectively and continue leading a vibrant, fulfilling life. Embrace this journey with the knowledge that aging brings wisdom, strength, and a renewed sense of self.

SEEKING SUPPORT

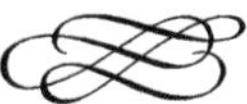

THE IMPORTANCE OF SUPPORT

Because this transition comprises physical, emotional, and psychological changes, having a strong support system is important for several reasons:

- Emotional stability: With the mood swings, anxiety, and depression that come about, support from others can provide emotional stability and help women navigate these challenging emotions.
- Validation and understanding: Knowing that others are experiencing similar changes can be comforting. It helps in validating your feelings and lessens feelings of isolation.
- Information and resources: Support networks are a good source of information about managing symptoms, available treatments, and coping strategies.
- Encouragement and motivation: Encouragement from others can help you keep a positive outlook and motivate you to engage in self-care practices and make lifestyle changes.

What Different Forms of Support Can Look Like

Support during menopause can come in various forms, each offering unique benefits. Here are some key types of support:

Social Support From Neighbors or Friends

Neighbors and friends can be an immediate and accessible source of support. They can offer

- Companionship: Regular social interactions that can help alleviate feelings of loneliness.
- Shared activities: Participating in activities together, like walking, working out, or attending social events, can improve physical and mental well-being.
- Listening ear: Just having someone to talk to about your experiences can be incredibly cathartic.

Building a Community of Like-Minded Individuals

Creating or joining a community of women who are going through the same transition can be incredibly empowering. You can try

- Support groups: These can be in-person or online forums where you can share your experiences, challenges, and hacks.
- Workshops and seminars: Educational events focused on menopause can provide valuable information and foster a sense of community.
- Social media groups: Online platforms can offer a space for continuous support and information exchange.

Speaking to Family Members

Family members can play a role in providing support through

- Understanding and empathy: Teaching your family about menopause can foster understanding and empathy, minimizing misunderstandings and potential conflicts.
- Practical help: Your family can help with daily tasks, giving you some relief and more time to focus on self-care.
- Emotional support: A supportive family environment can reduce stress and improve emotional well-being.

The Health Benefits That Social Support Can Have

Having a robust support network can have health benefits, including:

Emotional and Psychological Health

- Reduced Stress and Anxiety: Social support can lower your stress levels and decrease feelings of anxiety, leading to better mental health.
- Improved Mood: Interacting with supportive people can boost your mood and reduce the risk of depression.
- Increased Self-Esteem: Feeling supported and understood can raise self-esteem and confidence.

Physical Health

- Better Sleep: Less stress and anxiety means improved sleep quality.
- Enhanced Immune Function: Social connections can strengthen the immune system, making your body more resilient against illness.
- Increased Longevity: Studies have shown that strong social networks are linked to longer life expectancy (Sifferlin, 2014).

Expressing Your Emotions in a Safe Space

Having a safe space to express your emotions is important during this time. It allows you to

- Process your feelings: Talking about your emotions can help you process and understand them better.
- Receive validation: Hearing that others have similar experiences can validate your feelings and lessen feelings of abnormality.
- Develop coping strategies: Sharing your experiences and coping strategies can open you to new insights and practical solutions.

Support during menopause is not just beneficial; it is essential. Whether it comes from friends, family, or a community of like-minded people, a strong support system can make a big difference in navigating this transition. The health benefits are quite profound, impacting both your emotional and physical well-being. So, fostering and seeking out support should be a priority.

ONLINE SUPPORT NETWORKS YOU CAN UTILIZE

The Benefits of Support Groups

Navigating menopause can be challenging for some, and many women find solace and strength in connecting with other women who are going through the same thing. Online support groups offer a unique platform for sharing experiences, finding resources, and getting much-needed emotional support. Here are some key benefits of using these networks:

Knowing You Aren't Alone

One of the most profound benefits of joining a support group is the realization that you are not alone. Menopause can feel isolating at times, especially if your symptoms are severe or if those around you don't fully understand what you're going through. Online support groups connect you with a community of women who share similar experiences, giving you some reassurance and reducing feelings of loneliness.

Find Coping Strategies

Support groups are a treasure trove of practical advice and coping strategies. Members share the things that have worked for them in managing symptoms. This collective wisdom can help you discover new methods that you otherwise may not have known to alleviate your symptoms and improve your quality of life.

Being Open About Emotions and Frank About Your Experiences

Menopause brings with it a rollercoaster of emotions. Support groups provide a safe space to express these feelings openly and honestly. Sharing your experiences and hearing others' stories can be therapeutic. It can help you process your emotions and gain some much-needed perspective. This openness fosters a sense of camaraderie and mutual understanding.

Gain Confidence

Engaging in a support group can significantly boost your confidence. Hearing from other women who have successfully navigated the transition can inspire and empower you. Also, discussing your symptoms and concerns in a supportive environment can help you feel more in control of your health and well-being.

Online Organizations You Can Get Involved With

There are a lot of reputable online organizations and support groups that provide valuable resources and a sense of community for women going through menopause. Here are some you can consider:

Red Hot Mamas Menopause Support Group

Red Hot Mamas is one of the largest menopause education programs in North America. Their online community offers a wealth of resources, including webinars, articles, and forums where you can connect with other women. They focus on providing evidence-based information and practical advice to help you manage your symptoms effectively.

Menopause and Me

Menopause and Me is an online platform that offers support and information tailored to the needs of women going through the transition. The website has articles, personal stories, and expert advice on a wide range of topics to do with menopause. Their forums allow you to ask questions and share experiences with other members.

"Friend for the Ride" Blog

"Friend for the Ride" is a blog that addresses the journey of menopause with humor and honesty. The blog features personal stories, tips, and interviews with experts. It offers a unique blend of support and information, helping you navigate the change with a more positive outlook.

Changes During the Change

Changes During the Change is a dedicated online community for women going through menopause. The site offers forums, chat rooms, and virtual meetups where you can connect with other women. It's a supportive space to discuss your experiences, ask questions, and find comfort in shared stories.

Endocrine Society Patient Engagement

The Endocrine Society provides a comprehensive resource hub for women going through menopause. Their website offers educational materials, patient guides, and links to support groups. The Endocrine Society's patient engagement initiatives are designed to empower women with knowledge and connect them with a broader community of support.

Online support networks play an important role in helping you navigate the complexities of menopause. You get a platform to share experiences, find practical advice, and get some emotional support. Joining these groups helps you realize that you are not alone, teaches you new coping strategies, lets you express your emotions openly, and gains the confidence to manage this transition the best way you can. Whether through established organizations like Red Hot Mamas or personal blogs like "Friend for the Ride," these communities offer invaluable support during this stage of life.

MANAGING MENOPAUSE AT WORK

Menopause can present unique challenges in the workplace, but with the right strategies and support, you can manage them effectively. Here, we will explore the importance of starting a conversation with your employer, practical solutions to make work more manageable, and the benefits of building a support network with colleagues, if possible.

Why It's Important to Start the Conversation

Opening up about menopause with your manager (if you have one) can feel uncomfortable, but it's an important step towards creating a supportive work environment. Effective communication leads to understanding, accommodation, and a healthier workplace environment.

How you can start the conversation:

- Ask for a private meeting: Set up a one-on-one meeting in a private room where you can speak openly without interruptions or distractions.

- Prepare what you are going to say and be constructive: Think about the key points you want to discuss. Explain how menopause is affecting your work and suggest ways your employer can help.
- Remember that your employer has a duty of care: Employers are obligated to support their employees' health and well-being. Don't forget that you are entitled to this support.
- Suggest regular check-ins: Propose regular follow-up meetings to discuss how things are going so you can adjust accommodations as needed.

Practical Solutions

Seeking support from your manager is just the first step. Make the effort to explore practical solutions and accommodations that can make your work life more manageable.

Symptoms like hot flashes, fatigue, and brain fog can impact performance. Identifying and requesting specific adjustments can help you manage these symptoms more effectively.

Things You Can Request to Make Work Easier

- Flexible working hours: Adjusting your work hours can help you manage symptoms that may be worse at certain times of the day.
- Temperature control: Ask for a fan, a cooler workspace, or permission to adjust the office thermostat.
- Access to rest areas: Having a quiet space where you can take short breaks can help you manage fatigue and stress.
- Ergonomic workstations: A comfortable workstation can alleviate physical discomfort.
- Remote work options: If possible, working from home can keep your stress levels down and provide a more comfortable environment to manage symptoms.

Building up a Support Network With Colleagues

Connecting with colleagues who may be experiencing similar challenges can provide invaluable emotional and practical support.

Benefits of a Support Network

- Knowing you aren't alone: Sharing experiences with others going through similar issues reduces feelings of isolation.
- Finding coping strategies: Exchanging tips and strategies helps you learn new ways to manage symptoms.
- Being open about emotions: Having a safe space to express your feelings can relieve stress and improve mental health.
- Gaining confidence: Support from colleagues can boost your confidence in managing menopause at work and advocating for your needs.

How to Build One

- Start Conversations: Be open about your experiences and encourage others to share theirs.
- Form a Group: Create a formal or informal support group at work.
- Share Resources: Exchange information about helpful resources, articles, and support services.
- Encourage Inclusivity: Make sure the group is welcoming to all who need it, fostering a culture of understanding and support.

Starting the conversation with your manager, thinking of practical solutions, and building a support network with colleagues lets you create a more manageable and positive work experience. Seeking and offering support is a sign of strength and resilience.

WHEN TO SEE A DOCTOR

Even though menopause is a natural phase, it can bring about symptoms that require medical attention. Knowing when to seek help is important for managing your health and well-being during this transition.

Many women can manage symptoms on their own, but seeing a doctor can provide some support and alternative treatment options. Consulting a professional can help you navigate the complexities of menopause, ensuring you receive the best possible care tailored to your specific needs.

When Is It Necessary?

- Extreme symptoms: If you experience severe symptoms that impact your daily life, like debilitating hot flashes, chronic insomnia, or intense mood swings, seek medical advice. These symptoms can often be managed with the right treatment.
- Unexpected symptoms: Sometimes, menopause can present unusual symptoms that may not be immediately recognized as related to hormonal changes. If you experience symptoms like heart palpitations, severe joint pain, or memory loss, consult a doctor to rule out other potential health issues.
- Experiencing vaginal bleeding after menopause: Any vaginal bleeding after menopause should be evaluated by a healthcare provider. It can be a sign of underlying conditions like endometrial hyperplasia or cancer, and prompt medical attention is necessary to determine the cause and appropriate treatment.

How Your Doctor Can Help You

When you seek medical advice, your doctor can offer a range of treatments and support to help you manage your health.

Your doctor will conduct a thorough evaluation, which could include discussing your symptoms, medical history, and a physical exam. This helps to identify the underlying causes of your symptoms and tailor a treatment plan specifically for you.

Treatment Options

Based on your evaluation, your doctor may suggest treatment options like:

- Hormone Replacement Therapy (HRT): HRT can help alleviate many symptoms by replacing the hormones that your body no longer produces. Your doctor can help you weigh the benefits and risks of HRT and determine if it is the right course of treatment for you.
- Non-Hormonal Treatments: There are several non-hormonal medications available that can help manage symptoms. Your doctor can prescribe these if HRT is not suitable for you.
- Lifestyle and Dietary Advice: Your doctor can provide guidance on lifestyle changes and dietary adjustments that can help reduce symptoms. This might include recommendations for exercise, stress management techniques, and nutritional supplements.
- Support for Mental Health: Menopause can affect mental health, leading to issues such as anxiety and depression. Your doctor can refer you to a mental health professional or suggest treatments like therapy or medication to support your mental well-being.

Ongoing Monitoring and Referrals to Specialists

Regular follow-up appointments with your doctor can help monitor your progress and make any necessary adjustments to your treatment plan. This ensures that you continue to receive effective care as your symptoms progress.

If needed, your doctor can refer you to specialists like gynecologists, endocrinologists, or mental health professionals for further evaluation and treatment.

Knowing when to seek medical help and understanding how your doctor can help you allows you to take proactive steps to manage your menopausal symptoms effectively. Remember, seeking medical advice is a positive and empowering decision that can enhance your quality of life during this time.

Support during menopause is a need, offering significant benefits that impact emotional and physical well-being. Emotional stability is crucial as support from others helps navigate mood swings, anxiety, and depression. Knowing others share similar experiences provides validation and reduces feelings of isolation. Support networks are invaluable sources of information on managing symptoms, treatments, and coping strategies, while encouragement from others can help maintain a positive outlook and motivate lifestyle changes. Social support provides companionship, practical help, and a listening ear. Building communities of like-minded individuals through support groups, workshops, and social media can foster understanding and empathy, alleviating loneliness and stress. The health benefits of strong social connections include reduced stress and anxiety, improved mood and self-esteem, better sleep, enhanced immune function, and increased longevity. Creating safe spaces to express emotions helps process feelings, receive validation, and develop coping strategies. Overall, a robust support system is vital for a smoother transition through menopause.

EMPOWER MORE WOMEN LIKE YOU!

Knowing you have control over your menopause experience is deeply empowering – and you can help to bring that power to more women.

Simply by sharing your honest opinion of this book and a little about how it has helped you, you'll help new readers find the guidance they're desperately searching for.

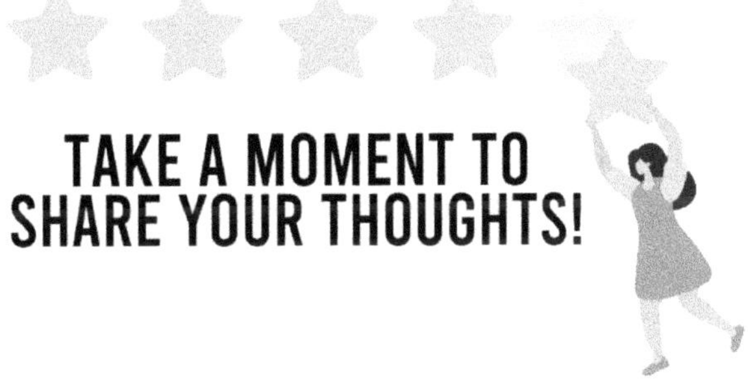

Thank you so much for your support. May your menopause be the start of an empowering transformation!

Scan the QR code below

CONCLUSION

Navigating through the complex and often challenging journey of menopause is no small feat. As we've explored throughout this book, understanding and managing menopause involves addressing a myriad of physical, emotional, and psychological changes. From the basics covered in Part 1: Menopause 101 to the more intricate aspects of side effects and symptoms in Part 2, and finally, the holistic approaches and support systems in Part 3, you've equipped yourself with a comprehensive toolkit.

Part 1: Menopause 101 laid the groundwork, providing a clear understanding of what menopause is and how it affects the body. We delved into the specifics of managing early menopause, recognizing that this earlier onset brings its unique challenges and considerations.

Part 2: Side Effects and Symptoms, we confronted the diverse range of symptoms that can accompany menopause. From handling hormonal mood swings and addressing sexual side effects to managing hair changes, sleep disruptions, cognitive shifts, and weight fluctuations, each chapter aimed to offer practical advice and solutions to help you cope with these often daunting changes.

Part 3: Natural Remedies and Resources emphasized the importance of a holistic approach to managing menopause. We explored alternative medicine and natural supplements, offering you various paths to alleviate symptoms. Moreover, recognizing the important role of support systems, we discussed seeking professional guidance and connecting with communities for emotional and psychological support.

By now, you are well-equipped with the knowledge and strategies to manage menopause with greater ease and confidence. It's important to remember that while you may not be able to completely eradicate the symptoms of menopause, you can certainly find ways to feel comfortable and confident in spite of them. The journey through menopause is unique for every woman, but with the right information and resources, you can navigate this transition more smoothly.

Armed with the insights from this book, you can move forward knowing that you have the tools to manage this phase of life. Embrace this transition with the understanding that while challenges will arise, they are manageable with the right approach. By combining medical advice, lifestyle adjustments, and support, you can make informed decisions that contribute to your well-being.

As you continue on your journey, remember that menopause is a natural phase of life, and with the knowledge and strategies you've gained, you can face it with resilience and grace. Your comfort, confidence, and overall health are within your control, and you are now better prepared to thrive during this transformative period.

GLOSSARY

- Androgen Decline in Aging Women (ADAW): The decrease in androgen hormone levels during menopause, affecting libido and overall well-being.
- Andropause: Often referred to as *male menopause*, it describes age-related changes in male hormone levels, particularly testosterone.
- Bioidentical Hormones: Hormones that are chemically identical to those the human body produces. They are often used in hormone replacement therapy.
- Bone Density: The amount of mineral matter per square centimeter of bone, often measured to assess the risk of osteoporosis.
- Climacteric: The period of life characterized by the transition from the reproductive phase to the non-reproductive state, encompassing perimenopause and menopause.
- DEXA Scan: Dual-energy X-ray absorptiometry, a test that measures bone mineral density to assess the risk of fractures and osteoporosis.
- Early Menopause: Menopause that occurs between the ages of 40 and 45, earlier than the typical onset.

- Estrogen: A primary female sex hormone responsible for the regulation of the menstrual cycle and reproductive system.
- Follicle-Stimulating Hormone (FSH): A hormone produced by the pituitary gland that stimulates the growth of ovarian follicles in women. Elevated levels can indicate menopause.
- Genitourinary Syndrome of Menopause (GSM): A term encompassing various vaginal and urinary symptoms associated with menopause, like dryness, irritation, and urinary incontinence
- Hormone Replacement Therapy (HRT): Treatment used to relieve symptoms of menopause by replenishing estrogen and, sometimes, progesterone levels.
- Hot Flashes: Sudden feelings of warmth, often intense, which are a common symptom of menopause.
- Hysterectomy: Surgical removal of the uterus, which can lead to surgical menopause if the ovaries are also removed.
- Menopausal Transition: Another term for perimenopause, indicating the gradual process leading up to menopause.
- Oophorectomy: Surgical removal of one or both ovaries, often resulting in surgical menopause.
- Osteopenia: Reduced bone density, often occurring during menopause due to hormonal changes.
- Osteoporosis: A condition characterized by weakened bones and an increased risk of fractures, commonly associated with decreased estrogen levels in menopause.
- Pelvic Organ Prolapse: The descent of pelvic organs (e.g., bladder, uterus) due to weakened pelvic floor muscles, which can be exacerbated by menopause.
- Perimenopause: The transitional phase before menopause when the body undergoes changes leading to menopause. Symptoms may begin while menstrual cycles are still regular.
- Post menopause: The phase of life after menopause, marked by the stopping of menstrual periods for 12 consecutive months.

- Premature Menopause: Menopause that occurs before the age of 40, either naturally or due to medical interventions.
- Progesterone: A hormone involved in the menstrual cycle, pregnancy, and embryogenesis. It works alongside estrogen.
- Selective Estrogen Receptor Modulators (SERMs): Compounds that act on estrogen receptors; they can mimic or block estrogen in different tissues.
- Surgical Menopause: Menopause induced by surgical removal of the ovaries (oophorectomy) or uterus (hysterectomy).
- Testosterone: While primarily known as a male hormone, it is also present in women and affects libido, energy, and bone strength.
- Vaginal Atrophy: Thinning, drying, and inflammation of the vaginal walls due to decreased estrogen levels, often resulting in discomfort and painful intercourse.
- Vasomotor Symptoms: Symptoms related to the regulation of blood vessel diameter, including hot flashes and night sweats.
- Weight-Bearing Exercise: Physical activity that forces you to work against gravity; important for maintaining bone density. Examples include walking, running, and strength training.

REFERENCES

Agarwal, Neha. "Menopause Quotes: A Beacon of Light Amid Change." Menoveda. Last modified November 6, 2023. https://menoveda.com/blogs/knowledge/menopause-quotes-a-beacon-of-light-amid-change

Arvind, D. S. S. (2023, May 2). *What are premenopause, perimenopause, and menopause?* ICliniq. https://www.icliniq.com/articles/womens-health/premenopause-peri menopause-and-menopause

Barhum, L. (2023, April 21). *Everything you need to know about menopause and sleep.* Verywell Health. https://www.verywellhealth.com/menopause-and-sleep-7376634

Barraclough, A. (2022, October 28). *Early menopause affects 5% of women: Here's how to know if you're at risk.* Marie Claire UK. https://www.marieclaire.co.uk/life/health-fitness/early-menopause-symptoms-734738

Black cohosh: Uses, side effects, interactions, dosage, and warning. (2019). Webmd. https://www.webmd.com/vitamins/ai/ingredientmono-857/black-cohosh

Blasi, J. (2024, March 6). *Can brain fog be caused by vitamin deficiency?* Dr Jenna Blasi. https://drjennablasi.com/brain-fog-vitamin-deficiency/

Body composition: Fitness explained. (2023, May 3). Atlas Bar. https://atlasbars.com/blogs/fitness-explained/body-composition-fitness-explained

Boskey, E. (2024, January 4). *Sex after menopause.* Verywell Health. https://www.very wellhealth.com/sex-after-menopause-5185098

Breathing exercises for asthma. (n.d.). Allergy Asthma Network. https://allergyasthmanet work.org/news/breathing-exercises-for-asthma/

Brown, B. (2023, September 4). 12 most common causes of memory loss. *Forbes.* https://www.forbes.com/health/conditions/memory-loss/

Campbell, M. (2023, August 23). *How to build a support system for mental health and wellness.* Growth Tactics. https://www.growthtactics.net/how-to-build-a-support-system-for-mental-health-and-wellness/

Cherry, K. (2023, March 3). *How social support contributes to psychological health.* Verywell Mind. https://www.verywellmind.com/social-support-for-psychological-health-4119970

Chintapalli, S. (2022, July 22). *Red clover: 7 health benefits, uses, and side effects.* MedicineNet. https://www.medicinenet.com/red_clover_benefits_uses_and_side_effects/article.htm

Coping with the emotions of menopause. (n.d.). ET Healthworld. https://health.economic times.indiatimes.com/news/industry/coping-with-the-emotions-of-menopause/93571006

Davis, D. M., & Hayes, J. A. (2012, July). What are the benefits of mindfulness? *American Psychological Association.* https://www.apa.org/monitor/2012/07-08/ce-corner

Derwent, H. (2022, June 28). *Iron: Are you deficient?* Menopause Center. https://www.menopausecentre.com.au/iron-are-you-deficient

Dibiase, S. (2023, June 26). *Pelvic pain and cramping after menopause.* Pelvic Floor Pro. https://pelvicfloorpro.com/pelvic-pain-and-cramping-after-menopause/

The emotional challenges of experiencing early menopause. (2023, September 17). Neural World. https://www.neuralword.com/en/article/the-emotional-challenges-of-experiencing-early-menopause

Empowered intimacy: Navigating sexual health through menopause and beyond | midi. (2024, April 8). Midi. https://www.joinmidi.com/post/sexual-health-menopause

Evening primrose oil. (n.d.). NCCIH. https://www.nccih.nih.gov/health/evening-primrose-oil

Fleiss, C. (2022, August 15). *How to deal with menopause emotions?* Medindia. https://www.medindia.net/news/how-to-deal-with-menopause-emotions-208278-1.htm

Fraser, C. (2017, August 7). *8 upper-body stretches for when your back, neck and shoulders are sore and painful.* Live Love Fruit. https://livelovefruit.com/8-upper-body-stretches-for-painful-back-neck-shoulders/

Garcia, M. (2023, November 3). *Anguish meaning: What does anguish feel like and how to deal.* Mind Journal. https://themindsjournal.com/anguish-meaning/

George, C. (2023, May 17). *How to have healthy, shiny silky hair.* Wiki How. https://www.wikihow.com/Have-Healthy-Shiny-Silky-Hair

Hickle, J. (2022, July 7). *How do I stop menopause irritability?* TimesMojo. https://www.timesmojo.com/how-do-i-stop-menopause-irritability/

Houry, A. (2024, January 22). *How support groups can help after a cancer diagnosis.* Hematology and Oncology Associates of Northern California. https://hoaonc.com/how-support-groups-can-help-after-a-cancer-diagnosis/

How to take valerian: A comprehensive guide. (2023, November 11). Neuralworld. https://www.neuralword.com/en/article/how-to-take-valerian-a-comprehensive-guide-3

Impact of menopause on women's hair: Understanding changes and care strategies - brightenyourmood.com. (2024, April 30). Brighten Your Mood. https://www.brightenyourmood.com/impact-of-menopause-on-womens-hair-understanding-changes-and-care-strategies

Kahn, J. (2024, February 17). *Why menopause causes sleep problems and what to do about it.* Rise Science. https://www.risescience.com/blog/menopause-sleep-problems

Lee, E. (2022, August 26). *What is early menopause?* CPD Online College. https://cpdonline.co.uk/knowledge-base/care/early-menopause/

Manaher, S. (2024, February 20). *Analgesic vs cinchophen: When to use each of them?* Grammar Beast. https://grammarbeast.com/analgesic-vs-cinchophen/

Martin, A. (2022, September 22). *Where to buy black cohosh plants?* IHomeRank. https://www.ihomerank.com/article/where-to-buy-black-cohosh-plants

Martin, H. (2022, July 4). *How the menopause affects women's sleep - and five tips to help you.* Talented Ladies Club. https://www.talentedladiesclub.com/articles/how-the-menopause-affects-womens-sleep-and-five-tips-to-help-you/

Mastering emotional regulation strategies. (2023, December 19). ESoft Skills. https://esoftskills.com/emotional-regulation/

Menopause. (2019, December 12). Wikipedia; Wikimedia Foundation. https://en.wikipedia.org/wiki/Menopause

Menopause and sex. (n.d.). Gransnet. https://www.gransnet.com/health/sex-and-the-menopause

Menopause and sex: Everything you need to know. (2022, August 4). Foria. https://www.foriawellness.com/blogs/learn/menopause-and-sex

Menopause self-care strategies every woman should know. (2023, July 13). Nuzzie. https://nuzzie.com/blogs/cozy-corner/menopause-self-care-strategies-every-woman-should-know?pb=0

Navigating menopause: A comprehensive guide to embracing change. (2023, May 23). Bosque Women's Care; Bosquewomenscare. https://www.bosquewomenscare.com/post/navigating-menopause-a-comprehensive-guide-to-embracing-change

Navigating menopause: A guide for women. (2023, September 15). Neural World. https://www.neuralword.com/en/article/navigating-menopause-a-guide-for-women

Navigating menopause: Understanding mood swings, changes, and concerns. (2024, February 22). Hati Health. https://www.hati.health/post/navigating-menopause-understanding-mood-swings-changes-and-concerns

Navigating menopause: Understanding the transition and managing symptoms. (2023, September 11). News Directory 3. https://www.newsdirectory3.com/navigating-menopause-understanding-the-transition-and-managing-symptoms/

Nazish, N. (2018, January 17). 10 simple ways to start eating healthier this year. *Forbes.* https://www.forbes.com/sites/nomanazish/2018/01/09/10-simple-ways-to-start-eating-healthier-this-year/

Nersisyan, A. (2024, April 7). *Signs that perimenopause is ending: Key indicators.* Docus. https://docus.ai/symptoms-guide/signs-perimenopause-is-ending

Noble, D. (2023, November 21). *When your ovaries check out early: Early menopause.* Mayo Clinic Press. https://mcpress.mayoclinic.org/women-health/when-your-ovaries-check-out-early-early-menopause-2/

Office of dietary supplements - Black Cohosh. (2020, June 3). NIH. https://ods.od.nih.gov/factsheets/BlackCohosh-HealthProfessional/

Pacheco, D. (2021, January 22). *How can menopause affect sleep?* Sleep Foundation. https://www.sleepfoundation.org/women-sleep/menopause-and-sleep

Painful intercourse: When to seek medical help for UTI, exer's guide for timely treatment. (2023, August 2). Exer Urgent Care. https://exerurgentcare.com/resources/painful-intercourse-when-to-seek-medical-help-for-uti-guide-to-timely-treatment/

Reinfeld, D. J. (2022, June 2). *Menopause and sleep, link, causes and remedies.* Mantra Care. https://mantracare.org/therapy/sleep/menopause-and-sleep/

Russell, L. (2016, August 12). *Journey through the menopause.* Chantry Health. https://www.chantryhealth.com/journey-through-the-menopause/

Savvas, M. (2020, November 16). *Sleep problems and the menopause.* Total Health. https://www.totalhealth.co.uk/clinical-experts/mr-michael-savvas/sleep-problems-and-menopause

Schimelpfening, N. (2003, February 21). *The 5 major classes of antidepressants.* Verywell Mind; Verywellmind. https://www.verywellmind.com/what-are-the-major-classes-of-antidepressants-1065086

Sharer, H. (2023, January 15). *What is healthy body composition? Exploring how diet, exercise, genetics, stress, and more impact your health - the enlightened mindset*. The Enlightened Mindset. https://www.tffn.net/what-characterizes-healthy-body-composition/

Sharp, L. (2024, February 5). *Navigating menopause: A holistic approach to women's health at serenity osteopathy*. Serenity Osteopathy. https://www.serenityosteopathy.co.uk/post/navigating-menopause-a-holistic-approach-to-women-s-health-at-serenity-osteopathy

Sheppard, L. (2024, May 14). *Best ways to navigate the emotional shifts of menopause*. Paperblog. https://en.paperblog.com/best-ways-to-navigate-the-emotional-shifts-of-menopause-7781198/

Shkodzik, K. (2022, December 19). *The 34 symptoms of menopause + 5 treatments*. Mira Care. https://www.miracare.com/blog/what-are-the-34-symptoms-of-menopause/

Sizensky, V., & Berman, N. (2016, December 14). *How your vagina changes in midlife*. Healthy Women. https://www.healthywomen.org/content/article/how-your-vagina-changes-midlife

Social support system - better psychological health | montare. (2020, October 26). Montare Behavioral Health. https://montarebehavioralhealth.com/blog/social-support-system/

St. John's wort: Uses, side effects, interactions, dosage, and warning. (2017). Webmd. https://www.webmd.com/vitamins/ai/ingredientmono-329/st-johns-wort

Support system: How family and friends shape our lives. (2024, April 19). FasterCapital. https://fastercapital.com/content/Support-System--How-Family-and-Friends-Shape-our-Lives.html

Szymanowski, J. (2023, May 2). *Can pre-workout kill you? (Serious risks explained)*. Torokhtiy. https://torokhtiy.com/blogs/guides/can-pre-workout-kill-you

Ten exercises to strengthen lower back | Know exercises for lower back pain. (n.d.). Metropolis India Lab. https://www.metropolisindia.com/blog/preventive-healthcare/exercises-for-a-strong-lower-back

Thirty adoption counselor interview questions and answers. (2023, October 17). InterviewPrep. https://interviewprep.org/adoption-counselor-interview-questions/

Transitioning to independent living for young adults with disabilities. (2023, December 30). ESoft Skills. https://esoftskills.com/transitioning-to-independent-living-for-young-adults-with-disabilities/

Turner, L. (2021, June 30). *9 nutrients for balanced neurotransmitters*. Clean Eating. https://www.cleaneatingmag.com/clean-diet/general-health/9-nutrients-for-balanced-neurotransmitters/?scope=anon

Vatcher, A. (2023, September 25). *The remarkable benefits of breathing: A path to health and well-being*. Calgary Therapy Institute. https://www.calgarytherapyinstitute.com/post/the-remarkable-benefits-of-breathing-a-path-to-health-and-well-being

Wankhade, N. (2023, August 2). *Body composition analysis*. HealthifyMe. https://www.healthifyme.com/blog/body-composition-analysis/

Wellme menorescue reviews (urgent warning!) do not buy until knowing the truth! (2023, November 15). Bellevue Reporter. https://www.bellevuereporter.com/blog/wellme-menorescue-reviews-urgent-warning-do-not-buy-until-knowing-the-truth/

What's the best menopause specialist? MSCP is the answer! (2023, September 11). Pandia Health. https://www.pandiahealth.com/blog/whats-the-best-menopause-specialist/

Wulf, S. (2023, August 30). *17 astonishing facts about Cimicifuga*. Facts. https://facts.net/nature/plants/17-astonishing-facts-about-cimicifuga/